AYURVEDA & AROMATHERAPY

The Earth Essential Guide to Ancient Wisdom *and* Modern Healing

DR. LIGHT MILLER, ND

and

DR. BRYAN MILLER, DC

LOTUS

This book is not intended to treat, diagnose or prescribe. The information contained herein is in no way to be considered as a substitute for your own inner guidance, or consultation with a duly licensed health care professional.

Cover design, page design, composition and indexing by Paul Bond, Art & Soul Design
Editing by Susan Tinkle
Illustrations by Peter Sinclair, Jessica N. Miller and Jancis Salerno
Cover photograph by Mary Murphey, September Image Inc.
Photographs by Laszlo Photography

2nd printing 1999
First printing 1995

Printed in the United States of America

Library of Congress Cataloging-in-Publication Data
Miller, Light and Bryan,
    Ayurveda and Aromatherapy: The Earth Essential Guide to Ancient
       Wisdom and Modern Healing / by Light and Bryan Miller
    includes bibliographical references and index.
    ISBN 13: 978-0-9149-5520-7   ISBN 10: 0-9149-5520-9
                                                    95-80409
                                                    CIP

Published in 1995 by
Lotus Press, P.O. Box 325, Twin Lakes, Wisconsin 53181
Website: www.lotuspress.com   E-mail: lotuspress@lotuspress.com

ACKNOWLEDGEMENTS

Bryan

To my parents for their love and support in becoming who I am.
To my sisters Julie and Peggy for being who they are.

To Liz Thorpe who set me on my metaphysical journey, Don Crosby,
Father Yod, Dr. Ted Morse, Dr. Stober, Dr. G. Morris Ellison, Dr. James Hattaway,
Dr. Robert Sherman and all who have assisted me on the path.

Thanks to Dr. Lad, Dr. Chopra, Dr. Frawley and Dr. Svoboda for their
pioneering work in bringing Ayurveda to recognition in this country.

To my sons, Bodhie and Cedar, who help me let go of my attachments,
and my dear wife (who leads me into expansion).

Light

Special thanks to Lenny Blank (Lennyji) for his trust, love and support;
to Michael and Mary Murphey—her divine energy kept pouring into
every interaction of this book; to Lehsa Orcutt for taking time to
work with us in transcribing and sharing her love.

My thanks to Dr. David Bigden for his knowledge and support; to Alan Breslow
for his inspiration and organization; to Charlene Knopp for taking over
a difficult project; to Peter Sinclair, Jessica N. Miller and Jancis Salerno
for their delightful illustrations.
To Sunny Greenberg and Jennifer Copeland for their loving support.
To Selby Botanical Gardens for allowing us to share their beautiful space.

To our staff, Carmela and Joy, who kept things running so we could take time
to write; to my friend Alicia Bjerke, for sharing the vision of
Earth Essentials and supporting me in my work; to Sandy Levy and Duane
O'Kane for helping with the vision of the Holy Relationship; to Raam Panday
for bringing me back to my roots in Ayurveda and Kaya Kalpa.

To all the teachers of Ayurvedic medicine,
especially my 110-year-young teacher, Dr. Chotay.

To Victoria Edwards for being a pioneer of aromatherapy in this country;
to all the people who are committed to the growth of essential oils
in this country, and all those who cross my path and are open
to receive knowledge.

I dedicate this book to my grandmother

for her wonderful knowledge of the herbs,

to my children

who allow me to experiment with their bodies

in the use of essential oils, herbs and diet.

TABLE OF CONTENTS

FOREWORD

When I was asked to write a foreword for "Ayurveda and Aromatherapy," I agreed immediately, based on knowing the Millers for the last two years. As we make our way through this life, on occasion we are fortunate enough to cross paths with others whose integrity and desire to improve the human experience is exceeded only by their love and genuine caring. Light and Bryan Miller exemplify the best of such high-minded people. I wholeheartedly support their healing and educational work and know that their intent is for personal, community and planetary transformation. I feel honored to have been asked to write this foreword.

Life is filled with circumstances that call for choices to be made. Some are insignificant and can be made with little or no effort, while others impact our lives in a big way, demanding study and soul-searching before a decision is made. Obviously, choosing what color car you will drive pales in importance when compared to choosing where to raise your children or what kind of work you will do.

At the top of the list of importance, when it comes to making choices, are the ones you make regarding your health. Let's face it, when it comes right down to it, nothing is more important than your health. And making the right choices can determine how long you will live and how healthfully.

We are facing a health care crisis in America today. Two out of three people are overweight, our expensive medical system has no cure for 80% of disease, and contributes to the causation of 10% of all illness with inappropriately applied drugs and surgery. Heart disease and cancer, the major causes of death in this country, are largely preventable by diet, exercise and life style changes; people don't need more, expensive, health care, they need a deeper understanding of how to eat, exercise and live in balance with natural cycles and laws.

I immediately noticed some significant similarities between "Nature Hygiene" and "Ayurveda."

1. Toxemia (ama) is recognized as a major cause of congestion, blockage and disease. It begins with poor digestion, then spreads to cause problems in other parts of the body and must be removed in order to build health.

2. The Kapha diet and lifestyle closely matches the "Fit for Life Regimen," cleaning out excess waste, helping with weight normalization and providing a boost of energy with its abundance of fresh fruits and vegetables.

3. Natural hygiene and Ayurveda both recognize natural cycles of appropriation (Pitta-digestion), assimilation (Kapha-building up tissue) and elimination (Vata-movement) which occur daily. It is important to eat when digestion is strongest, rest when the body is assimilating and respect (support) the period of elimination.

Additionally, Ayurveda's emphasis on taking responsibility for self care, preparing your own food, appropriate exercise, eating seasonally and maintaining a positive state of mind, are all congruent with my understanding of human health.

My experience with aromatherapy includes the use of essential oils for environmental fragrancing and therapeutic inhalations for a temporary sinus infection. Most intriguing for me are the connections between smell, emotions and states of mind. Imagine assisting human growth, development and transformation using natural plant extracts. The Millers' book demonstrates numerous methods to use essential oils for self healing.

Both sciences, Ayurveda and aromatherapy, offer hope for the healing of mankind, and this book is a huge contribution to their joining. The book's step-by-step, self diagnoses of metabolic types and "how to use" format make it easy for the western mind to understand and apply these important healing modalities.

Harvey Diamond

Co-author of *Fit for Life*, #1 on the New York Times best seller list for forty consecutive weeks, with worldwide sales of ten million copies. Author of the forthcoming book *You Can Prevent Breast Cancer*.

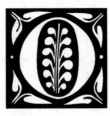nce upon a time,
when the earth was young...

... THERE WAS A KINGDOM of happiness and health, where all the people lived in connectedness with each other and the earth. The arts flourished; everyone sang and played musical instruments, and received satisfaction by perfecting their skills and talents. Each adult in the kingdom practiced a profession that supported the community, while also giving them joy. Free time was spent in self-study, play and artistic expression.

Children were revered and everyone cared for them. As they grew, they were taught about the world around them. They saw that everything was a lesson; a gift. Every plant and animal had a part in the cycles of nature; every experience was an opportunity for growth. The children were carefully watched, and encouraged in the arts and the life skills where they showed natural ability and passion. Because they were raised with love and respect, it reflected in their gentle treatment of one another. The older children took special care of their younger friends. Learning and play were one and the same.

The forests of the kingdom were carefully managed, and tended in such a way that the animals were undisturbed by the selective gathering of lumber, herbs and firewood. Forest guardians carefully chose old or damaged trees for harvest, thus the ecological balance was maintained. Herbs were gathered in a way that ensured that there was always plenty of every species.

The farmers took great joy in caring for their fields and plants. Human waste was considered a treasure, to be carefully collected by each family and transported back to the farming districts to be composted, returning its richness to the soil. The spreading of leftover straw from the harvest, and periodic flooding of the fields, made weeding unnecessary, and all the land was rich and fertile. Fruits and vegetables were traded in central market places for needed goods or services.

The marketplace was filled with beautiful arts and crafts. The people entertained each other in the streets and homes with spontaneous music, song, dance and plays. Athletics were encouraged—swimming, running, gymnastics, archery and all games. The people were strong, brave and happy.

A special group of healers (a combination of doctors, chemists and holymen), prepared perfumes, medicines, incense, herbal wines and oils. Special plants, roots, flowers, barks and resins were gathered and skillfully distilled or prepared. Beautiful aromas permeated every facet of life. Healing was easily accomplished, due to the power of the plant essences, insightful application by the healers, and the inherent wholeness of the way of life.

The people were presided over by a king whose training was in the benevolent management of the resources and the people he served. He was educated and counselled by holy men whose connectedness and wisdom ensured the tranquility of the kingdom. Although the kingdom was self-suf-ficient, the king encouraged an exchange of goods and culture from neigh-boring kingdoms. Peace and happiness were the kingdom's greatest export. Life was sweet and all was good. May the kingdom be restored.

THE ENLIGHTENED PRACTICE OF HEALING

Three patients sit in a doctor's reception. Each suffers from arthritis, yet each is different. The first patient, a tall, thin woman, is the first to see the doctor. As she gets up from the chair, her joints crack; she moves to the examining room in obvious pain and stiffness. After examining the patient and taking her case history, the physician prescribes moist heat, a detoxify-ing diet, and massage with medicated sesame oil. Special attention is given to cleansing the colon with daily castor oil and herbs. After one week, the patient is placed on a diet which restricts the use of fresh fruits and vegetables and is high in dairy products and rich oily foods.

The second patient is a ruddy-faced gentlemen of medium build, who appears to be slightly overheated in a room where everyone else is comfortable. Herbs to calm the digestion are prescribed. A special diet of cooling foods and cold compresses is recommended for his painful joints. His diet includes lots of fresh fruits, vegetables and sweet foods, with restrictions on proteins, oils and fermented dairy products.

The third patient, a large-framed, slightly overweight woman, moves steadily into the doctor's office on legs that are markedly swollen and edematous (holding water). The doctor prescribes spicy herbs to stimulate the digestion, heating essential oils mixed with alcohol to be massaged into her swollen joints, and a diet in which sugar, dairy and oily foods are strictly avoided.

How could this possibly be? How could three patients with the same disease be treated in such a varied and seemingly contradictory fashion? It is because the physician practices Ayurveda. He doesn't see three cases of arthritis, he sees three metabolically different people who are all having difficulty with their joints; each with a different set of symptoms and each needing a very different type of treatment.

SECTION I

AYURVEDA: THE SCIENCE OF LIFE

5

CHAPTER ONE

HISTORY AND PHILOSOPHY

Ayurveda is the world's oldest recorded healing system. Used for 5,000 years by many thousands of doctors on millions of patients, it is a proven system of prevention and healing. Ayurveda's goal is to achieve health by working toward balance and harmony, not by fighting disease. Prevention is emphasized over cure. Ayurveda recognizes the importance of physical balance, emotional release, mental health, environmental mindfulness and spiritual progression in the total health picture. Ayurveda is the only system of medicine which recognizes ten different metabolic types.

Western medicine does very well in cases of traumatic injury, acute and emergency care. But we in the West suffer more from auto-immune diseases such as arthritis, allergies, heart disease, cancer and even addiction. Because Ayurveda is an all-inclusive body of knowledge which uses a low-tech approach to healing, it is a system that can be adapted to all peoples and climates. Using natural forces such as heat, cold, light, herbs, foods, minerals, exercise and working with the mind and emotions through meditation, Ayurveda may be the basis of a global medicine, accessible and affordable to all.

Ayurveda is the current rage in alternative medicine, with thousands of people flocking to hear best-selling author Deepak Chopra, M.D., and visiting Ayurvedic clinics around the world. Ayurveda has several levels of treatment. At its most basic level, patients are able to treat themselves with simple diet and lifestyle changes, assisted by an understanding of their metabolic type and their own inherent strengths and weaknesses. Essential oils can be a powerful component of self treatment.

The purpose of this section is to give the reader a basic understanding of Ayurveda and how it can be used to bring balance and restore health. To discover your metabolic type, and in which direction you may be imbalanced, fill in the questionnaire on pages 25-29. There are also many books listed in the bibliography which we recommend for a more detailed study of Ayurveda. If you are not already a student of Ayurveda, our hope is that this will be an introduction into an exciting new world of self-healing and discovery.

HISTORY

Ayurveda was discovered and developed by ancient Indian holy men known as "Rishis." Due to their relationship (connectedness) to both the spiritual and physical worlds, they were able to discern the basic nature of the universe and man's place in it. They developed an oral tradition of knowledge that was fluid and allowed for growth. As new therapies and herbs were discovered and trade brought new information from other cultures, Ayurveda was built. The Rishis were scientists who made huge advances in the fields of surgery, herbal medicine, the medicinal effects of

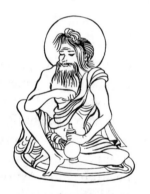

Rishi

minerals and metals, exercise, physiology, human anatomy, and psychology. Their surgeries included difficult procedures such as Caesarean section (successfully performed in the West only in the last 100 years). Passed down from teacher to student for centuries, this information was recorded when written language was developed: the Rig Veda (4500 years ago), the Atharva Veda, (3200 years ago) and others.

As knowledge of Ayurveda spread to other civilizations, its adaptability was recognized and it was often integrated into local forms of medicine.

Ayurveda had a profound effect on the medicine of Tibet, China, Persia, Egypt, Greece, Rome, and Indonesia.

Ayurvedic medicine was suppressed in India during British colonial rule. In 1833, the East India Company closed and banned all Ayurvedic colleges. For almost 100 years, Ayurveda was known as "the poor man's medicine," practiced only in rural areas where western medicine was too expensive or unavailable.

With India's independence, Ayurveda has re-emerged to gain equal footing with "Western Medicine." Currently, 70% of India's population is treated Ayurvedically. In 1978, at a conference on Third World Medicine sponsored by the World Health Organization (WHO) of the United Nations, it was concluded that Ayurveda would be the best system of medicine for undeveloped countries. There is hope that a global medicine will be created with Ayurveda as its base; its low cost, use of local herbs and remedies, adaptability to any climate, and reduced dependence on pharmaceutical products, are all favorable aspects for the world's population. Western, Chinese and traditional native medicines may be appropriately blended in each locale.

PHILOSOPHY

Ayurvedic theory believes that health results from harmony within one's self. To be healthy, harmony must exist between your purpose for being, your thoughts, your feelings, and your physical actions. Your purpose is peaceful, yet if your thoughts are fearful and your emotions negative, your physical body will manifest some dis-ease as a "wake-up call to change." In Ayurveda, the manifestation of disease is actually considered to be a good sign, because it reveals a previously hidden aspect of oneself... an aspect to be healed. Health is harmony within all aspects of self. This inner harmony also becomes manifest as harmony with family, friends, co-workers, society, and nature.

Often the first questions an Ayurvedic physician may ask are: "What is your purpose in life? And what is its appropriate form (work, job, activity, etc.)? How are your relationships?" When harmony exists in these areas, physical healing is so much easier.

The goal of Ayurveda is true freedom from death and disease; enjoyment of uninterrupted physical, mental, and spiritual happiness and fulfillment. It may sound surprising, but according to Ayurvedic philosophy, enjoyment is one of life's purposes. But you can lose your ability to enjoy if you overindulge, and disease is one of nature's ways of saying you've overindulged. Either you limit yourself or mother nature will limit you. We have more degenerative disease in the West because of our abundance and tendency to overindulge.

Ayurveda's Four Goals in Life

1. The fulfillment of your duties to society.
2. The accumulation of possessions while fulfilling duties.
3. Satisfying legitimate desires with the assistance of one's possessions.
4. The realization that there is more to life than duties, possessions and desires.

Ayurvedic philosophy believes that only a person with a strong immune system can be healthy. The practitioners identify the immune system as a fragment of nature (the Divine Mother). This gift from her creates us, sustains us, nourishes us, and protects us from outside invasion. As long as our immune system is strong, we suffer no disease. The ancient vedic word for immunity means "forgiveness of disease"—from the concept that negative thoughts

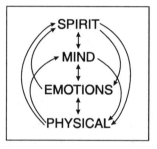

Fully Integrated Being

and lifestyles cause disease. Disease, therefore, is a message about a need for change... if only we can understand this. In this sense, strength comes from transforming our projections about our symptoms. Healing comes from seeing adversity as a challenge, by taking back our negative thoughts about people and events. We can transform disease into a "perfect opportunity." Spiritual health, then, is a dynamic balance between a strongly integrated individual personality and nature (a nature that's understood to encompass all aspects of existence). This is only possible when people remember their debt to nature.

In summary: Ayurveda believes that health results from the relationship (the connectedness) between self, personality, and everything that goes into our mental, emotional, psychic, and spiritual being. It believes that health also results from good relations with others, from an acknowledged indebtedness to mother nature, from the realization of one's purpose, and from the pursuit of legitimate goals in life. Ayurvedic philosophy maintains the importance of a strong immune system, that forgiveness is strengthening, and that immortality is possible.

THE FIVE ELEMENT THEORY

According to the Five Element Theory, the human being is a small model of the universe. What exists in the human body exists in altered form in the universal body. Ayurveda believes that everything is made up of five elements, or building blocks: earth, water, fire, air, and ether. Their properties are important in understanding balances and imbalances in the human body.

Earth is representative of the solid state of matter; it manifests stability, fixity and rigidity. We see around us rocks and soil standing against the wearing forces of water and wind. Our body also manifests this earth/solid-state structure: bones, cells and tissue are physical structures through which our blood courses and oxygen is transported. Earth is considered a stable substance.

Water characterizes change. In the outer world we see water moving through its cycles of evaporation/clouds/condensation/rain, we see it moving around solid matter such as rocks and mountains, and we see it eventually wearing away solid, immovable matter as it flows from the mountains to the sea. We see rivers carrying dissolved soil and nutrients, carrying economic trade and exchange of information and culture—we see the earth's bodies of water nurturing life everywhere. Our blood, lymph, and other fluids move between our cells and through our vessels, bringing energy, carrying away wastes, regulating temperature, bringing disease fighters, and carrying hormonal information from one area to another. Water is considered a substance without stability.

 Fire is the power to transform solids to liquids, to gas, and back again. The heat of the sun melts ice into water that becomes vapor under its influence. Fire provides power to the water and weather cycles of nature. The sun's energy is the initiator of all energy cycles on earth—including all food chains. Within our bodies it is fire (energy) that binds the atoms of our molecules together; that converts food to fat (stored energy) and muscle; that turns (burns) food into energy; that creates the impulses of nervous reactions, our feelings, and even our thought processes. Fire is considered form without substance.

 Air is the gaseous form of matter which is mobile and dynamic. We do not see the air that blows through the tree's leaves, but we feel it. We know how material it can be—how it can respond to energy, absorb it, and give it off—when we watch or experience a hurricane, typhoon or tornado. We feel air as it courses down our throats and into our lungs—cut that off for more than a few minutes and we know with our whole being how fundamental air is to life. Within the body, air (oxygen) is the basis for all energy transfer reactions—oxidation. Clean and pure, it is a key element required for fire to burn. Air is existence without form.

 Ether is the space in which everything happens. Like outer space with millions of miles between celestial bodies, or the inner space of our bodies where our very atoms are only .00001 charged particle and .99999 emptiness. Space, the distance between things—that which helps to define one thing from another. Ether is only the distances which separate matter.

THE THREE DOSHAS

In Ayurvedic philosophy, the five elements combine in pairs to form three dynamic forces (interactions) called doshas. Dosha means "that which changes" because doshas are constantly moving in dynamic balance, one with the others. Doshas are primary life forces or biological humors. They are only found in life forms (similar to the concepts of organic chemistry), and their dynamism is what makes life happen.

The five elements combine to create the three doshas (forces)

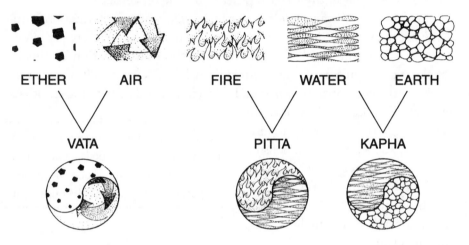

ETHER   AIR   FIRE   WATER   EARTH

VATA   PITTA   KAPHA

Vata (va-ta) is a force conceptually made up of the elements ether and air. The proportions of ether and air determine how active Vata is. The amount of ether (space) affects the ability of air to gain momentum, as expressed in Vata. In the body, Vata is movement (a dynamism of the combination between ether and air), and manifests itself in living things as the movement of nerve impulses, air, blood, food, waste and thoughts.

When the movement of air is unrestricted by space (as in the open ocean) it can gain momentum to become hurricane winds moving at speeds of over 150 mph. When air is restrained in a box, it cannot move and becomes stale.

Vata has seven characteristics, which are: cold, light, irregular, mobile, rarefied, dry, and rough. These qualities characterize their effect on the body. Too much Vata force can cause nerve irritation, high blood pressure, gas and confusion. Too little Vata, we have nerve loss, congestion, constipation and thoughtlessness.

 Pitta (pit-ta) is a force conceptually created by the dynamic interplay of water and fire. These two seemingly opposed forces represent transformation. They cannot change into each other, but they modulate each other and are vitally necessary to each other in the life processes.

In our bodies Pitta is manifested by the quality of transformation. Pitta is the enzymes which digest our food and the hormones which regulate our metabolism. In our mind, the Pitta force is the transformation of chemical/electrical impulses into understood thoughts. Too much Pitta can cause ulcers, hormonal imbalance, irritated skin (acne), and consuming emotions (anger). Too little Pitta and we have indigestion, inability to understand, and sluggish metabolism.

The Pitta force is described according to eight characteristics which affect the body: hot, light, fluid, subtle, sharp, malodorous, soft and clear.

> When you boil water on a fire, if the fire is too hot, all the water boils away and the pot burns. If you put too much water into the pot, it overflows and puts out the fire.

 Kapha (ka-fa) is the conceptual equilibrium of water and earth. Kapha is structure and lubrication—it draws on the conceptual characteristics of the elements of earth and water. At one level, Kapha is the cells which make up our organs and the fluids which nourish and protect them.

In the Ayurvedic organization of cause and effect, too much Kapha force causes mucous buildup in the sinus and nasal passages, the lungs and colon. In the mind it creates rigidity, a fixation of thought, inflexibility. Not enough

> When a handful of sand is thrown into a container of water, the two will separate as the sand settles to the bottom. Only by continuous stirring will the mixture remain in balance.
> The force of Kapha is like the stirring, maintaining the balance.

Kapha force causes the body to experience a dry respiratory tract, burning stomach (due to lack of mucous, which gives protection from excess stomach acids), and inability to concentrate. Kapha force is expressed according to the following qualities: oily, cold, heavy, stable, dense and smooth.

Changing Forces

These three dynamic forces are constantly changing and balancing each other in all living things. They make life happen. In a plant, Vata is concentrated in the flowers and leaves (which reach farthest out into space and air), Kapha is concentrated in the roots (where water is stored in the embrace of earth), and Pitta is found in the plants' essential oils, resins and sap (especially in spices which stimulate digestion). Different plants have different concentrations of V-

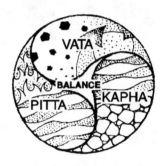

Changing Forces

P-K (Vata, Pitta, Kapha). We can use different foods, plants, and specific plant parts to alter our body's proportion of V-P-K. Eating root vegetables, milk products, or sedating herbs like valerian, increases our Kapha. Drinking herbal flowers like jasmine, or eating dry grains, increases our Vata forces. Eating hot, spicy foods like cayenne, or concentrated protein like bee pollen, increases our Pitta tendencies.

Climatic Influences

The climates we live in and the change of seasons also add or subtract from our V-P-K balance. Hot summers or hot climates increase our Pitta. Dry climates or cold autumn winds increase Vata. Wet winters and damp climates add to Kapha.

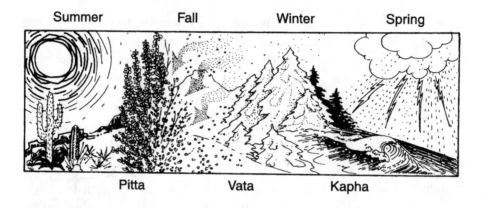

Summer   Fall   Winter   Spring

Pitta   Vata   Kapha

Life Stages

The stage of life we are in also affects V-P-K balance. The increase in the substance of the body which occurs during childhood growth means that Kapha forces are dominant during this cycle of life. The hormone changes which transform us into adults indicate that our early and middle years are under Pitta influences. As we age, we can shrink and dry out, indicating an increase of Vata forces.

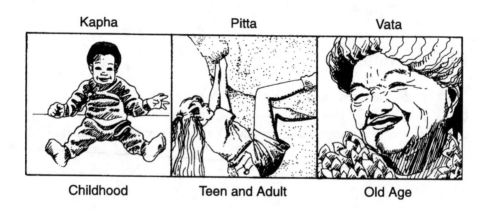

Kapha   Pitta   Vata

Childhood   Teen and Adult   Old Age

Ayurvedic Cycles of the Day
as told by Jean-Pierre LeBlanc (of Aroma Joy, B.C., Canada)

Kapha I Cycle 6:00 a.m. - 10:00 a.m.
All movements slow down. If you sleep past 6:00 a.m. it's harder to get up and you feel groggy. Food eaten now will not digest as well and should be light.

Pitta I Cycle 10:00 a.m. - 2:00 p.m.
Your metabolism gears up to its highest at 12:00 noon. This is the best time to eat your largest or most concentrated meal and take vitamins for greatest absorption.

Vata I Cycle 2:00 p.m. - 6:00 p.m.
A time of increased movement and activity. Your evening meal should be lighter than lunch. Mental activity and conversation should be lively.

Kapha II Cycle 6:00 p.m. - 10:00 p.m.
The energy slows down for bed and rest. Sleep will come easily and quickly. If you don't go to sleep by 10:00 p.m., you may toss and turn, especially if you eat late.

Pitta II Cycle 10:00 p.m. - 2:00 a.m.
Time of active, colorful dreams and deep sleep. If you happen to stay up, your metabolism may get geared up for a late night snack and activities, which you will regret the next day.

Vata II Cycle 2:00 a.m. - 6:00 a.m.
Corresponds to the ascending universal currents which are used by meditators to achieve high spiritual states. If you wake up at 4:00 or 5:00 a.m. and do spiritual exercise it will stay with you all day long as focused energy. If you sleep past 6:00 a.m., you fall into lethargic Kapha time.

Repeat Cycle

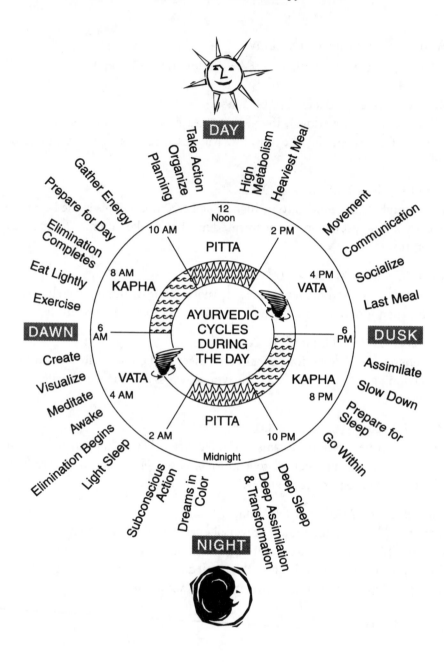

Ayurvedic Cycles of the Day

CHAPTER TWO

INDIVIDUAL BALANCE AND BODY TYPES

*E*ach of us is born with a unique bal-ance of V-P-K that makes us who we are and determines our strengths and weaknesses. No two people are the same, but there are said to be three pure types and seven mixed types (this type-ing is used for the sake of evaluation and treatment). For example, a person born with a high proportion of Pitta and small amounts of

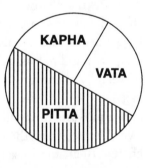

Vata and Kapha would be said to be a Pitta-dominant individual. Compare this Ayur-vedic view of the individual patient to our West-ern medical system where everyone is treated the same.

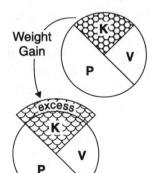

Weight Gain

Due to climatic, seasonal, life stage, diet or lifestyle changes, over time we may get out of balance. If we gained 30 lbs., our new V-P-K would change. Then we wouldn't feel "our-selves" until we return to the V-P-K combina-

tion we were born with. Ayurveda can help individuals discover their original balance and return to it.

VATA-DOMINANT TYPE

An individual with a primarily Vata influence will exhibit many of the following characteristics: they will have
a thin-framed body, whether tall or short; their joints
crack easily, and irregularity is the rule, including possible protruding joints, bow legs, disproportionate bodies
with long legs and short waist, scoliosis and uneven facial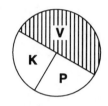
structure (deviated septum and crooked nose, etc.). If they do gain weight it
will be around the middle. Their skin will have a tendency to be dry, rough
and cool to the touch. Their skin coloration will be darker than the rest of
the family. Their hair may be dark, dry and kinky. Teeth are often crooked,
protruded with spaces and tendency toward receded gums. Their eyes can be
small, dry, active, black or brown. Appetite is often variable or low, although
when distracted, they will often skip meals and become ravenous, loading up
their plate with more than they could possibly eat. Their fingers and toes are
long and thin with nails which are brittle and crack easily. If they become
sick, pain and nervous disorders are likely. Their thirst is variable and their
bowel movements are often gassy, dry, hard and constipated. They are physi-
cally active, but expend their energy easily and may rely on caffeine, sugar
and stimulants to continue. Their mind is restless, active, curious and creative. Under stress they can become fearful, insecure and anxious. They
change their mind easily, have good short-term memory but forget easily.
They often dream about flying, running, jumping and fear. Their sleep is
difficult, interrupted and they can experience insomnia. Their speech is fast,
chaotic, impulsive and they often talk with their hands. Money goes through
their hands quickly as they spend impulsively. Their pulse is thready, feeble
and erratic. Vata predominant types will vary greatly from one to another,
but will share many of the above characteristics.

PITTA-DOMINANT TYPE

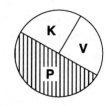

An individual who is primarily Pitta will have a moderate frame that demonstrates good proportions. They can gain or lose weight relatively easily. Their skin is often delicate, oily, burns easily, with a coppery or yellowish tone and is warm to the touch. Freckles and moles are common with a tendency to acne. They perspire readily. Their hair is soft, blond or red, grays early with tendency to early thinning or balding. Fingers are well formed and proportional. Fingernail beds have a pink appearance. Eyes are sharp, penetrating, gray, green, with a yellowish tint to the sclera (whites). If they become ill they will experience fever, inflammation and infection. They are often thirsty. Their bowel movements are soft, oily and loose, three times a day or more. They enjoy moderate activity and love competition due to their aggressive nature. They are intelligent and determined with a sharp memory. Under stress they can be irritable, driving, angry and jealous. Dreams are fiery, passionate and colorful. Their sleep is moderate and sound. Speech is sharp, clear, fluid and can be cutting and sarcastic. Pittas spend moderately and methodically. Their pulse is strong and regular. You can often tell a Pitta by their passion, high directed energy and their commitment.

KAPHA-DOMINANT TYPE

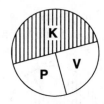

The pure Kapha is easy to recognize; large bodies on large frames. The Hawaiians are a Kapha people. Their skin is thick (3/4" on forearm), oily, cool to the touch, pale and lighter than others in their family. They perspire moderately. They gain weight easily and must exercise to lose it. Their hair is thick, oily, wavy with thick eyebrows and lashes. Teeth are strong, white, large and well formed. Eyes are big and attractive. Appetite is slow and steady, although they can easily skip meals without effect. If Kaphas become ill, congestion, excess mucous and water retention are common. They rarely experience thirst. Bowel movements are thick, oily, and regular (once a day). Peaceful and content, they move slowly and waste little energy. Endurance is good. Negative tendencies may be self centered-ness, greed and over sensitivity. They are steady, loyal friends and employees. Slow to learn new things, they seldom forget anything once learned. Dreams are often romantic and involve water. Their speech is slow and monotonous or melodious. They spend slowly, save easily and always have full cupboards. Their pulse is slow and steady.

THE SEVEN MIXED TYPES

In India, where people largely marry into their own tribe or group, single-dosha types predominate. In the West, we are a mixing pot; for the most part everyone is able to marry as they wish, and so mixed types predominate. Usually, in a mixed type, one dosha will be dominant, with a second dosha being a close second. For example, a Vata-Pitta person will have more and stronger Vata tendencies than Pitta. A Pitta-Vata person will have more Pitta qualities. Finally, there's the type called balanced tri-dosha (V-P-K), where no one type is predominant.

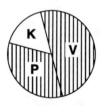

VATA-PITTA (V-P) are thin, like a pure Vata-type, quick moving, friendly, talkative, but more enterprising and sharper of intellect. They don't have the extremes of Vata, and are not as high-strung or irregular. They have stronger digestion and greater tolerance to cold. They are more tolerant of noise and physical discomforts. They have the strong drive of Pitta with the imagination of a Vata-type. They can easily fall into patterns of addiction and need stability.

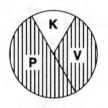

PITTA-VATA (P-V) are of more medium build with more musculature than V-Ps. They're also quick in movement, have good stamina, are often assertive, with obvious intensity, but with a Vata-type's lightness. They have strong digestion and more regular elimination than V-P or V. If they are under stress, they can react with fear or anger which can make them insecure, tense and hard driven. They love to eat, have a good memory and are fluid speakers. Too much heat can bother them.

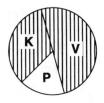

VATA-KAPHA (V-K) is often hard to identify with a questionnaire due to the presence of opposites in many characteristics, and Vata's indecisiveness. They often have a thin Vata frame with a Kapha-like relaxed, easy-going manner. They will be even-tempered unless stressed. Often quick and efficient, they are aware of their Kapha tendency to procrastinate. They desire to store up and save, and strongly dislike the cold. They can have slow or irregular digestion.

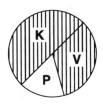

KAPHA-VATA (K-V) are similar to a V-K but are more solidly built and slower moving. They are even-tempered and even more relaxed that V-Ks, but with less enthusiasm. They tend to be athletic, with greater stamina. They may also have digestive irregularities, complain of cold, and suffer mucous buildup.

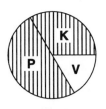

PITTA-KAPHA (P-K) have Pitta intensity in a strong Kapha body. They are more muscular than a K-type, and may be quite bulky. Their personality exhibits a K-type stability, with Pitta force and a tendency toward anger and criticism. They are a good type for athletes, having energy and endurance. They never miss a meal. They have Pitta-type digestion and Kapha-type resistance to disease.

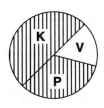

KAPHA-PITTA (K-P) are people who have a Kapha structure, but more fat than a P-K type. They are rounder in the face and body, move more slowly, and are more relaxed than P-Ks. They have a steady energy and even more endurance than a P or P-K type. They like exercise but are less motivated to do it than a P-K. They can be arrogant and unresponsive to criticism.

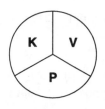

VATA-PITTA-KAPHA (V-P-K) are the hardest to describe, because they have equal amounts of each dosha. They are the most balanced with a tendency to long life, good health and immunity. Ayurvedic physicians say that these types are the most difficult to treat when they do get out of balance. There are very few true V-P-K types. People who think they are V-P-K are usually a two-dosha mixed type.

WHO AM I?

In studying the ten preceding body types and looking at yourself, remember that you are unique, and that this is an opportunity to learn about yourself. The following questionnaire will allow you to find out the V-P-K balance of your birth.

Body Type Questionnaire

On each line check the statement which best describes you. Occasionally, more than one statement will best describe you, or none.

Part I - Characteristics Which Do Not Change. The choices that you make here reveal your original metabolic type. This is the body type with which you were born, and how you were meant to experience the world. Of course, lifestyle, diet, climate, etc. can and will shift you from this (see Part II, characteristics which change), but the result will be compromised immunity and health. The distribution of your answers may reveal you to be predominately one type or a mixed type, and this basic configuration is where your health lies. Remember your numbers here and compare them to your Part II configuration.

Part I-Characteristics Which Do Not Change

Vata	Pitta	Kapha
☐ 1. Thin and unusually tall or short.	☐ 1. Medium body.	☐ 1. Large body.
☐ 2. Light, small bones and/or prominent joints.	☐ 2. Medium bone structure.	☐ 2. Heavy bone structure.
☐ 3. Long tapering fingers and toes.	☐ 3. Fingers and toes medium in length.	☐ 3. Fingers and toes short and squarish.
☐ 4. Thin as a child.	☐ 4. Medium build as a child.	☐ 4. Large or chunky as a child.
☐ 5. If gains weight, around middle.	☐ 5. If gains weight, deposits fat evenly.	☐ 5. Tends to gain weight, especially in rear and thighs.
☐ 6. Dark complexion (relative to family—tans easily).	☐ 6. Fair skin, sunburns easily, freckles and moles common.	☐ 6. Tans evenly.
☐ 7. Body hair scanty or overabundant, tends to be dark, coarse and curly.	☐ 7. Light body hair - fine texture.	☐ 7. Moderate amount of body hair.
☐ 8. Small forehead.	☐ 8. Medium forehead with folds and lines.	☐ 8. Large forehead.
☐ 9. Small, dark, active eyes.	☐ 9. Medium size, light green, gray, amber or blue eyes.	☐ 9. Large, liquid, sometimes blue, often chocolate brown eyes.
☐ 10. Crooked, uneven or buck teeth that are sensitive to heat and cold, may have needed braces.	☐ 10. Even teeth, of medium size.	☐ 10. Large, even, gleaming teeth.
☐ 11. Neck small, unsteady.	☐ 11. Moderate neck.	☐ 11. Large, steady neck.

Vata	Pitta	Kapha
☐ 12. Delicate chin.	☐ 12. Moderate chin.	☐ 12. Large jaw.
☐ 13. As a child, hair kinky, curly.	☐ 13. As a child, hair fine, light.	☐ 13. As a child, hair wavy & thick.

_____Total VATA   _____Total PITTA   _____Total KAPHA

Part II - Characteristics Which Change. This shows where your balance is now. Total your VPK here and compare it to your original VPK to see how you've shifted. Many of these characteristics are symptoms of imbalance and you may wish to be free of them. Example, if you were born primarily Vata, but in Part II demonstrate a shift into Kapha symptoms like weight gain, fluid retention, craving sweets, this shows a Kapha imbalance that needs correcting.

Part II - Characteristics Which Change

Vata	Pitta	Kapha
☐ 1. Difficulty gaining weight.	☐ 1. Can gain or lose weight if puts mind to it.	☐ 1. Gains weight easily, hard time losing without exercise.
☐ 2. Cold hands and feet.	☐ 2. Skin warm to touch.	☐ 2. Skin cool but not cold.
☐ 3. Dry skin (¼" thick - pinch skin on forearm), chaps easily. Prone to corns and callouses.	☐ 3. Oily skin, prone to pimples and rashes (¼ "- ½" thick).	☐ 3. Thick skin (¾+" thick), well lubricated.
☐ 4. Often suffers cracked, chapped lips	☐ 4. Deep, red lips, tendency toward cold sores, fever blisters.	☐ 4. Full, moist lips.

26

Vata	Pitta	Kapha
☐ 5. Dry hair, luster-less, split ends, dark, rough, wiry or kinky.	☐ 5. Fine, light, oily, blonde, red or early gray hair, early thinning or bald-ness possible.	☐ 5. Thick, slightly wavy hair, a little oily, dark, brown, lustrous.
☐ 6. Dislikes dryness and cold (likes warmth).	☐ 6. Prefers cool, well-ventilated places (dislikes heat).	☐ 6. Tolerates most climates (dislikes humidity).
☐ 7. Tongue dry with thin, grayish coating.	☐ 7. Tongue coating yellowish, orange or reddish.	☐ 7. Tongue swollen with thick, curdy, white coating.
☐ 8. Eyes often dry and scratchy, sclera (whites of eye) grayish or bluish.	☐ 8. Sclera has reddish or yellow tinge.	☐ 8. Tendency toward eye puffiness.
☐ 9. Bowel movement can be irregular, hard, dry or constipated.	☐ 9. Bowels loose - more than twice a day/diarrhea.	☐ 9. Large full bowel movement, once a day/mucous, itch-ing.
☐10. If ill: nervous dis-orders, sharp pain likely.	☐10. If ill: fevers, rashes or inflamation likely.	☐10. If ill: swelling, fluid retention, mucous, congestion.
☐11. Sexual interest variable, fantasy life active.	☐11. Highly sexed, arouses easily.	☐11. Steady sex, slow to arouse.
☐12. Menses irregular, scanty flow, severe painful cramps.	☐12. May bleed heavily, and long loose stool accompanies period.	☐12. Prone to water weight during menses, slight cramps, if any.
☐13. Either indulges in rich food or on strict diet.	☐13. Loves proteins, caf-feines & hot, spicy, & salty foods.	☐13. Loves sweets, dairy, bread and pastry.
☐14. Receding gums.	☐14. Inflamed, bleeding gums.	☐14. Thick gums.
☐15. Joints - painful, unsteady, crack-ing or stiff.	☐15. Joints - hot, swollen, burning.	☐15. Joints - loose, ach-ing, watery, swollen.
_____Total VATA	_____Total PITTA	_____Total KAPHA

27

Part III - The Mind. The mind of each metabolic type demonstrates favorable and unfavorable characteristics. Vatas are creative thinkers but change their mind often. Pittas have good memory and organization skills but can tend toward snap decisions and running over people in their drive to get things done. Kaphas work well with routine and follow directions thoughtfully but are slow to make decisions and can lack creativity. Knowing yourself and understanding how you think can save you much discomfort. For example, if your questionnaire reveals that you have predominately Vata mind characteristics you will be much happier in a job using your creativity rather than management or repetitive routines.

Part III - Mind

Vata	Pitta	Kapha
☐1. Concentration is short, short-term memory good, but forgets quickly.	☐1. Good short- and long-term memory, logical, rational thoughts.	☐1. Takes time to learn things, once learned, never forgets.
☐2. Dislikes routine.	☐2. Enjoy planning & organizing, especially if self-created.	☐2. Works well with routine.
☐3. Difficulty deciding, changes mind easily.	☐3. Rapid decision-making, sees things clearly.	☐3. Takes time making decisions, sticks with it.
☐4. Restless, active, likes movement.	☐4. Aggressive, likes competitive activities.	☐4. Calm, likes to relax, leisure activities.
☐5. Creative thinker.	☐5. Organized thinker.	☐5. Prefers to follow a plan or idea.
☐6. Does many projects all at once.	☐6. Constantly organizing, likes to proceed in orderly fashion.	☐6. Resists change, new projects; likes simplicity.
☐7. Knows a lot of people, few close friends.	☐7. Very selective, but creates warm friendships/makes enemies easily.	☐7. Loyal, with many friends.
☐8. Spends impulsively, money is to be used.	☐8. Plans spending, money is for achieving purpose.	☐8. Spends reluctantly, likes to save.
_____ Total VATA	_____ Total PITTA	_____ Total KAPHA

Part IV - The Emotions. The emotional characteristics of each type have positive and negative aspects. Vata people become easily anxious or fearful, yet can forget quickly and don't often hold a grudge. Pitta's anger comes quickly, but they have the ability to transform it to competitiveness or overcoming a challenge. Kapha's sensitivity means a slight is not easily forgiven, but that sensitivity makes them loyal and romantic.

Look at your choices in this section and note where you are emotionally: are you manifesting positive or negative aspects; are your emotions in line with your initial type (Part I), current balance (Part III) or have you developed characteristics outside of your dosha (summary of questionnaire, page 30).

Part IV - The Emotions

Vata	Pitta	Kapha
☐ 1. Experiences fear.	☐ 1. Experiences hate.	☐ 1. Experiences apathy.
☐ 2. Practices secretiveness.	☐ 2. Can be vindictive.	☐ 2. Can be uncaring.
☐ 3. Can be self-destructive.	☐ 3. Can be destructive.	☐ 3. Feels victimized.
☐ 4. Anxious.	☐ 4. Irritable.	☐ 4. Attached.
☐ 5. Sneaky.	☐ 5. Manipulative.	☐ 5. Greedy.
☐ 6. Nervous.	☐ 6. Angry.	☐ 6. Desirous.
☐ 7. Dynamic.	☐ 7. Perceptive.	☐ 7. Harmonious.
☐ 8. Communicative.	☐ 8. Caring.	☐ 8. Devoted.
☐ 9. Flexible.	☐ 9. Tolerant.	☐ 9. Patient.
☐ 10. Feelings and emotions change easily.	☐ 10. Aggressive about opinions and feelings, gives opinions even if they are not asked for.	☐ 10. Avoids giving opinions in difficult situations.
☐ 11. Dreams about flying, restless, nightmares.	☐ 11. Dreams in color, fast, passion, conflicts.	☐ 11. Romantic, short dreams, often involve water.
_____ Total VATA	_____ Total PITTA	_____ Total KAPHA

SUMMARY OF QUESTIONNAIRE

Part I shows where we began constitutionally and where we may need to return to feel "ourselves." Part II shows our immediate state of balance and makes us aware of symptoms that we may wish to see changed; this section will be your guide in choosing a lifestyle regime and diet to reduce your most aggravated dosha. Part III shows our mind's strengths and weaknesses. Understanding our mental nature can help us choose work which suits our innate abilities, and avoid those activities (occupations) which do not suit us. Part IV - if our negative or destructive emotions match our "Dosha Imbalance" (Part II), they will be taken care of by the appropriate diet and lifestyle regime (found in Chapter Four). If they fall out of pattern and are associated with a different dosha, specific essential oils to reduce those emotions can be used.

Totals Parts II, III & IV

_____Total VATA   _____Total PITTA   _____Total KAPHA

This three-part total shows where you are operating in body, mind and emotion at this moment. After initiating therapies, diet, and lifestyle changes to balance your doshas, you can retake these parts and see a shift. Part I will always remain the same and so is not included in the total nor retaken.

PULSE

The doshas (Vata, Pitta, Kapha), constantly adjust one against the others due to changes in our thoughts, feelings and actions. Our pulse reflects these changes, and we can detect imbalances before they manifest as a condition or disease. We are able to take action to create balance quickly.

Although good Ayurvedic practitioners do not rely on the pulse alone and will often ignore it if there seems to be conflict with other diagnostic findings, pulse diagnosis can be helpful in monitoring immediate conditions and establishing a rapport with the patient. By taking your own pulse at different times of the day (as it changes), you can develop sensitivity and skill.

Nature of Pulse

The general nature of the pulse is more important than any other aspect of pulse diagnosis. Vata pulse is fast (80-100 beats per minute), irregular, thready, said to be like a snake or leech. Pitta pulse is moderate (65-80 beats per minute), bounding, perky, wiry, jumpy and regular; compared to movement of a frog or a sparrow. Kapha is even, slow, languorous, wide, rolling, and its movement is compared to a swan, peacock or river (50-65 beats per minute).

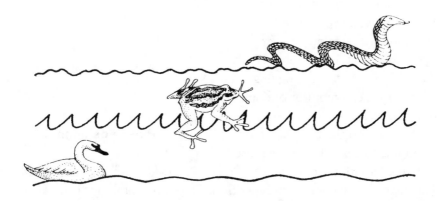

Three Pulse Waves

Times

For a neutral reading, it is best to take your pulse early, upon awakening, when you are calm and rested. After eating, exercise, sex, massage or hot bath, it may have a Pitta quality. After sleep or overeating, it may have a

Kapha quality. When anxious, nervous, tense, rushing or experiencing excessive change, your pulse can develop a Vata nature. Can you notice these influences on your pulse?

Positions

The pulse may be taken in many places on the body, but most commonly used and convenient is the radial pulse (thumb side) of the wrist. The pulse is taken on the right wrist of a man and the left wrist of a woman. With the wrist lightly flexed, place the index finger on first crease of the wrist. The middle and ring fingers are placed adjacent toward the elbow in the groove of the radial artery (see diagram). The pulse under the index finger indicates the general activity level of the Vata forces. The middle finger pulse indicates the general strength of the Pitta forces. The ring finger pulse is a general monitor of Kapha in the body.

Pulse Positions

Many people become frustrated if they cannot find the pulse or detect variations immediately. Practice anyway, with the calm assurance that the skill will come with repetition. Be positive and say "I think I feel a difference." Our western scientific minds demand an explanation on how things work before it will allow our intuitive feeling to take over.

Perhaps the best explanation of why pulse diagnosis works (along with tongue diagnosis, face diagnosis, foot reflexology, etc.) is the holotrophic theory of healing; it states that every part of the body is represented in every other part, similar to a hologram. In holographic photography, an image is made of an object; when light is projected through any part of that image, even the smallest fragment, the complete object appears in the projection. Similarly, any part of the body examined contains information about the complete body. We already know that every cell contains the complete blueprint of the body: DNA. Cloning takes one cell and replicates its entire source from that DNA fragment. Deepak Chopra, in his book *Quantum Healing*, describes how every cell has intelligent knowledge of our thoughts, feelings, and body conditions through a constant stream of information from our nervous impulses, hormones, and neurotransmitters. Dr. Chopra calls this the BODY-MIND—not separated, but unified by constant communication.

Pulse diagnosis can be one method through which a lay person can learn about his or her own body and the forces at play in differing conditions, times and situations.

CHAPTER THREE

THE TASTES OF LIFE

THE SIX TASTES

There are six tastes: sweet, sour, salty, pungent, bitter and astringent, and each is derived from two of the five elements. The tastes are important in seeing how "we are what we eat." Our bodies are formed by the elemental nature of our intake which increases or decreases doshic (VPK) balance.

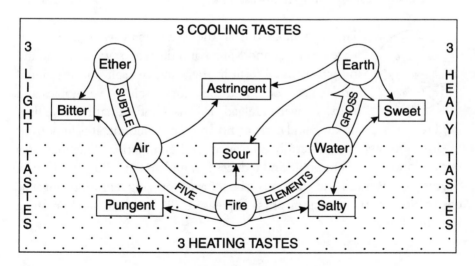

The Six Tastes and the Five Elements

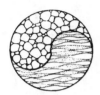 **Sweet** is made from the elements earth and water; it increases Kapha (also made from earth and water), and decreases Pitta and Vata. Sweet is found in sugars, carbohydrates, fats, oils and amino acids. Its characteristics are heavy, cold, and oily. While it builds tissue, it also can block ducts and channels, and its cold nature dampens the digestive fire. Over-indulgence in the "sweetness of life" produces Kapha illnesses such as obesity, diabetes, blocked circulation, indigestion, and respiratory congestion. On the emotional level, sweet provides satisfaction unless over-consumed, where it causes complacency and laziness and feeds greed and dissatisfaction (when sweets ferment they turn sour).

 Sour is created from the elements earth and fire. It increases Pitta and Kapha but decreases Vata. Sour is found in acid fruits (sour), acid vegetables (ascorbic acid), alcohol (oxalic acid), fermented products, cultured dairy products (lactic acid), and to a lesser extent, proteins (amino acids) and oils (fatty acids). Its properties are heavy, hot and oily. It strengthens digestive fire, and is contraindicated in gastritis, ulcers, inflammation, wasting, and other Pitta disturbances. It stimulates appetite and digestion, increases waste elimination, and reduces spasms. Sour is associated with envy, jealousy and dissatisfaction; the opposite of sweet. "Sour grapes" metaphorically refers to desire turning to distaste.

 Salty is composed from the elements of water and fire. It increases Pitta and Kapha and decreases Vata. It is found in concentrated form in rock salt, sea salt and in diluted forms in sea foods and the mineral salts in vegetables and fruits. If over-indulged, it causes inflammation, swelling, fluid retention, wrinkling and early aging. In proper amounts it is important in digestion, appetite, electrolyte balance, and elimination. Salt increases our zest and enjoyment of life and reduces fear and anxiety. But the effect of overuse on the mind and emotions is hedonism—craving sensation, anger at obstruction to indulgence or physical pleasure (like an "old salt" on leave from his ship).

Pungent is formed from the elements fire and air, and increases Pitta and Vata while reducing Kapha. Pungent is characteristically heating, light, and dry, and is found in spices and concentrated in essential oils (volatiles and aromatics). Pungent functions to stimulate secretions and digestive enzymes, increase appetite and metabolism. It is a treatment for Kapha disorders (obesity, stagnant circulation, diabetes, coughs, respiratory congestion), and aids in the elimination through the skin. Used in excess, it causes or increases pain, thirst, burning, impotence, faintness and debility. Mentally and emotionally, it creates extroversion and the need for stimulation, and increases irritability and anger.

Bitter is created by the elements air and ether. It increases Vata (air and ether) and decreases Pitta and Kapha. It is cooling, light and dry, and is found in bitter green-leafy vegetables (dandelion and endive), bitter herbs (golden seal and gentian), and bitter roots (turmeric). At normal consumption, it purifies and dries secretions, tones and tightens tissue. It is helpful for decreased appetite, digestive problems, fever, liver and skin irritations. Over-indulgence can cause all Vata disorders, including nerve irritations, weight loss, dryness, cracking skin, and lack of secretions. Emotionally, it produces dissatisfaction and realization of the need to change ("the bitter truth"). It reduces anger and complacency, but in excess can produce bitter obstinance, frustration, grief and insecurity.

Astringent is composed of the elements air and earth. It increases Vata and decreases Pitta and Kapha, because the air component overrides the earth influence. Astringent is found in tannins, barks, and resins (oak bark, myrrh) and astringent herbs and vegetables (beans, potatoes, alfalfa) and raw honey. In small amounts it reduces secretions, tightens and purifies body tissues. In excess it dries secretions and tissues causing constipation, thirst, tremors, and tingling. Emotionally, in overuse, it causes introversion, separateness, fear, and anxiety.

Summary of tastes

Through understanding taste and its influence on our doshic nature and metabolism, we can choose foods and essential oils to understand our cravings and emotions and balance ourselves. Western diet over-emphasizes sweet, sour and salty foods and produces a society which is greedy, indulgent, hedonistic and increasingly dissatisfied. A personal step toward change can be "tasting the bitter truth," looking inward and seeking balance through taste.

THERAPEUTIC USE OF TASTES

For people experiencing Vata excess:

Increase	Reduce
sweet	bitter
sour	astringent
salty	pungent

For people experiencing Pitta excess:

Increase	Reduce
sweet	salty
bitter	pungent
astringent	sour

For people experiencing Kapha excess:

Increase	Reduce
pungent	sour
bitter	salty
astringent	sweet

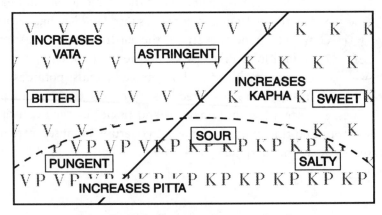

The Six Tastes and the Three Doshas

CHAPTER FOUR

THE SUBDOSHAS

*E*ach of the doshas, Vata, Pitta, Kapha, are forces acting in every part of the body, all the time. In the digestive tract, Vata creates the movement of food, Pitta is the digestive process which transforms the food into useable energy, and Kapha makes up the structures into which the food moves and into which the nutrients are absorbed. Even at the cellular level the three forces are in action, with Vata transporting nutrients into the cell, Pitta being the enzymes which allow the nutrients to be metabolized, and Kapha being the cell structure. Certain areas of the body have high concentrations of Vata, Pitta or Kapha and are said to be primary locations of the dosha. There are five concentrations of Pitta, Vata and Kapha, and each performs a different function.

Vata is concentrated in the brain, lungs, stomach, circulation and nervous sys-

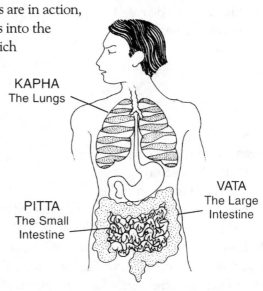

KAPHA
The Lungs

VATA
The Large
Intestine

PITTA
The Small
Intestine

Primary Sites of the Three Doshas

tem, with its greatest concentration in the colon. Pitta's primary concentration is in the small intestine, but also the liver, heart, eyes, and skin. Kapha has its primary location in the chest, but also the stomach, mouth, head and joints. When the doshas are out of balance, they will produce specific conditions which are characteristic of their location in the body.

The subdoshas are important in diagnosis and treatment. Even if you discovered that you are a pure fire-type with an imbalance of Pitta, during flu season you may experience a Kapha flu with an excess of mucous discharge. It would then be appropriate to drop your Pitta-reducing regimen, and use the essential oils that can reduce the aggravation of Kapha you are experiencing in your sinus area.

THE FIVE FORMS OF VATA

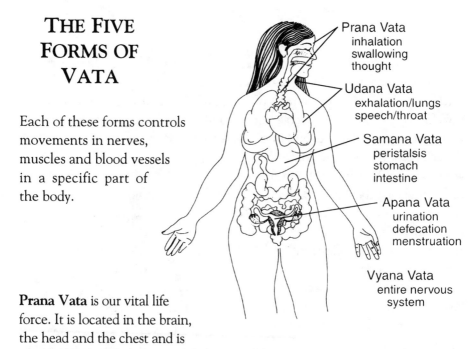

Prana Vata
inhalation
swallowing
thought

Udana Vata
exhalation/lungs
speech/throat

Samana Vata
peristalsis
stomach
intestine

Apana Vata
urination
defecation
menstruation

Vyana Vata
entire nervous
system

Each of these forms controls movements in nerves, muscles and blood vessels in a specific part of the body.

Prana Vata is our vital life force. It is located in the brain, the head and the chest and is responsible for inhalation and the downward movement, or swallowing, of food. It makes possible all of the senses, including the ability to think and have feelings. Almost all diseases have some aspect of disruption of the Prana Vata, and therefore breathing exercises and aromatherapy can be an important part in healing any condition. Our fast-paced society with its flood of impressions and over-stimulation causes us to unconsciously restrict our breathing and lowers our life force. Just notice how "dead" people appear as they watch TV; hardly breathing at all (thoroughly stimulated visually and auditorially, but hardly reacting).

Symptoms of Imbalance	Essential Oils to Restore Balance	Essential Oil Applications
worry	calamus	inhalations
anxiety	sandalwood	nasya (nose drops)
insomnia	rosemary	compresses
asthma	brahmi	seasonings in food
tension headaches	myrtle	and teas
hoarseness	hyssop	shirodhara
hiccups	basil krishna	
dry cough	angelica	
tuberculosis	cardamon	
shortness of breath	orange	
dehydration		
emaciation		
wasting		
poor memory		
senility		
irregular heartbeat	(see Section III for more information on	
loss of voice	oil applications and restoring balance)	

Udana Vata is concentrated in the lung and throat. It is known as the upward moving air and is responsible for exhalation. It makes speech possible, promotes physical strength, and creates a strong intellect and memory. Udana Vata allows the release of emotions and the letting go of thought projections (forgiveness).

Symptoms of Imbalance	Essential Oils to Restore Balance	Essential Oil Applications
dry eyes	chamomile	inhalations
sore throat	elecampane	compresses
tonsillitis	(inhalation only)	gargles
lack of enthusiasm	anise	
weakness	ajwan	

Symptoms of Imbalance (continued)
fatigue
earaches
speech defects
stuttering
cancer
over-excitement
dry cough

Samana Vata is responsible for moving food into the stomach and intestine by peristalsis. It is a balancer and equalizer of both the mind and the emotions. It is responsible for the movement of digested food into the metabolism.

Symptoms of Imbalances	Essential Oils to Restore Balance	Essential Oil Applications
too-slow or too-fast movement of food	ajwan	compresses
indigestion	cumin	food and drink
diarrhea	turmeric	seasonings
gas	ginger	
poor nutrition	basil	
low energy	cloves	
dehydration	nutmeg	
	dill	
	valerian	

Apana Vata, downward moving air, is responsible for excretion of urine, food residues, menstruation, ejaculation, and the birth process. It sustains the growth of the fetus. When Vata becomes imbalanced it will tend to collect here in the colon more than anywhere else in the body and is the primary site of excess Vata in the body.

Apana Vata (continued)

Symptoms of Imbalance	Essential Oils to Restore Balance	Essential Oil Applications
constipation	trifolia	compresses
diarrhea	ginger	basti (enema
diabetes	garlic	therapy)
menstrual disorders	cinnamon	douche
dysmenorrhea	lime	implants
sexual dysfunction	lemon	sitz baths
low back pain	onion	
stillbirth	parsley	
difficult birth	asafoetida	
	basil	

Vyana Vata is found throughout the body. Its force is distributed by the nervous system and the circulatory system. It moves nutrition into the cells and moves the waste out. It is responsible for perspiration, heart rhythm, constriction and dilation of the blood vessels, yawning, and the sense of touch. It is the force that moves any of the excess doshas into weaknesses or faults in the body.

Symptoms of Imbalance	Essential Oils to Restore Balance	Essential Oil Applications
joint-cracking	myrrh	baths
arthritis	camphor	massage lotions
nervousness	cardamon	food and drink
frequent blinking	cinnamon	
heart irregularity	eucalyptus	
poor circulation	valerian	
difficult body movement		

THE FIVE FORMS OF PITTA

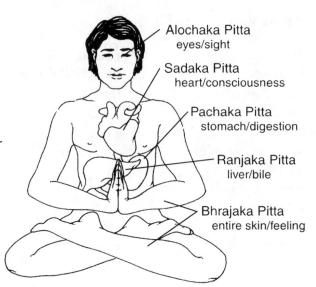

Alochaka Pitta
eyes/sight

Sadaka Pitta
heart/consciousness

Pachaka Pitta
stomach/digestion

Ranjaka Pitta
liver/bile

Bhrajaka Pitta
entire skin/feeling

The five forms of Pitta in the body are responsible for metabolism, digestion, enzymes, hormones, body chemistry, transformation, heat production, understanding of ideas, and vision.

Pachaka Pitta manifests as stomach acids and pancreatic enzymes. It produces appetite and cravings, breaks down food into nutrients and wastes and is the primary seat of Pitta. It is in this area that Pitta is most likely to accumulate and cause problems.

Symptoms of Imbalance	Essential Oils to Restore Balance	Essential Oil Applications
ulcers	coriander	food and drink additives
heartburn	cumin	stomach compresses
indigestion	turmeric	
addictions	fennel	
cravings	dill	
	peppermint	
	aloe vera (in fresh form, jel or juice—no essential oil exists)	

Ranjaka Pitta is active in the liver as bile, in the spleen as the production of red blood cells, and is responsible for maintaining blood chemistry, transforming food into metabolites and burning up the toxins that have accumulated in the blood.

Symptoms of Imbalance	Essential Oils to Restore Balance	Essential Oil Applications
anger	rose	food and drink additive
hostility	sandalwood	cool compresses
skin inflammations	chamomile	
liver disease	myrtle	
jaundice	lemon balm	
blood disorders	lavender	
anemia	coriander	
low blood pressure	neem	
	yarrow	
	chrysanthemum	
	turmeric	
	saffron	
	honeysuckle	

Sadaka Pitta is centered in the heart, and is regarded as the seat of consciousness. It brings contentment, courage, self reliance, clear-thinking, and digestion of thoughts.

Symptoms of Imbalance	Essential Oils to Restore Balance	Essential Oil Applications
heart attack	cardamon	heart compresses
indecision	rose	inhalations
emotional disturbance (anger, sadness, forgetfulness)	sandalwood	chakra anointment
	saffron	
	lotus	
	hina	
	gardenia	
	jasmine	

Alochaka Pitta is located in the eyes and is responsible for visual perception, the actual utilization of light by the body which directly stimulates the pineal gland.

Symptoms of Imbalance	Essential Oils to Restore Balance	Essential Oil Applications
eye diseases	camphor	cool compresses over eyelids (no essential oils should be put into the eyes, even in diluted form; however, floral waters (rose, myrtle) are appropriate for this use
visual problems	chrysanthemum	
red, irritated eyes	fennel	
anger		

Bhrajaka Pitta is located in the skin and is connected with our ability to feel what others feel (be objective). When it is in balance, our skin is radiant and glowing and when it is aggravated, it produces red, irritated skin.

Symptoms of Imbalance	Essential Oils to Restore Balance	Essential Oil Applications
acne	yarrow	massage oils and lotions
boils	chamomile	cool compresses
inflammation	peppermint	cool or slightly warm baths
rashes	coriander	
skin cancer	lavender	
all skin disorders	rose	

THE FIVE FORMS OF KAPHA

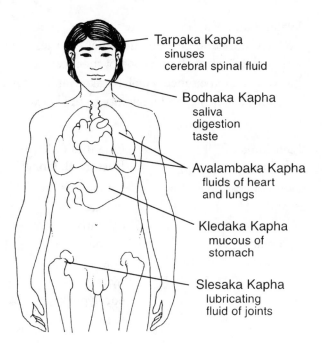

Tarpaka Kapha
sinuses
cerebral spinal fluid

Bodhaka Kapha
saliva
digestion
taste

Avalambaka Kapha
fluids of heart
and lungs

Kledaka Kapha
mucous of
stomach

Slesaka Kapha
lubricating
fluid of joints

The five Kaphas in the body are responsible for maintaining our tissues and structures, the fluids and lubrication, stability, firmness, flexibility and coolness in the body.

Bodhaka Kapha is found in the saliva and digestive fluids in the parotid gland. It is located in the mouth and is responsible for taste. Taste is particularly important to Kapha types and can result in overeating, achieving a dullness of taste and leading to imbalance. The first perception of life for a baby is the need for food, and in the first year of life, everything that the baby gets hold of goes immediately into the mouth: "oral fixation."

Symptoms of Imbalance	Essential Oils to Restore Balance	Essential Oil Applications
obesity	cardamon	mouthwash
food sensitivity	camphor	food and drink seasoning
congestion	calamus	
diabetes	fennel	
loss of taste	eucalyptus	
	ginger	
	myrrh	

Avalambaka Kapha is located in the heart and lining of the lung and provides lubrication for the movement of these very sensitive organs. A loss of these lubricating fluids is one of the most excruciating, painful conditions that you can experience. Avalambaka Kapha provides strength to the back, the chest, the heart, and flexibility to the body.

Symptoms of Imbalance	Essential Oils to Restore Balance	Essential Oil Applications
chest congestion	cardamon	inhalations
asthma	orange	compresses
lethargy	calamus	massage oil
back pains	elecampane	
stiffness	ginger	
	hyssop	
	eucalyptus	
	sage	

Kledaka Kapha is found in the stomach, and its mucous protects the stomach tissues from Pitta digestion. It mixes with the food and provides an internal lubrication.

Symptoms of Imbalance	Essential Oils to Restore Balance	Essential Oil Applications
slow digestion	ginger	compresses
fullness	ajwan	heating carminatives
excess mucous in the stomach	cinnamon	seasonings of food and drinks
	orange peel	
	oregano	
	thyme	
	cloves	

Slesaka Kapha lubricates the joints of the body and provides ease of movement. Aggravation or excess produces loose, swollen or watery joints.

Symptoms of Imbalance	Essential Oils to Restore Balance	Essential Oil Applications
loose joints	ginger	hot compresses
swelling	eucalyptus	massage oil (blends using mustard seed oil as a base)
stiffness	turmeric	
slow, painful movements	calamus	baths
	juniper	saunas
	cypress	

Tarpaka Kapha nourishes and sustains the sinuses, provides cerebral spinal fluid to cushion the brain and the spinal cord, and moistens the eyes and nose. It gives contentment and inner joy. In the state of enlightenment, tarpaka Kapha transforms itself to *amrita*, the nectar of immortality.

Symptoms of Imbalance	Essential Oils to Restore Balance	Essential Oil Applications
sinus irritation	basil	nasya
headaches	eucalyptus	inhalation
loss of smell	elecampane (inhalation only)	shirodhara
irritability	camphor	
	rosemary	

Subdoshas Symptom Survey

Use this chart to determine which subdoshas are out of balance.

VATA

Prana Vata

☐ worry
☐ anxiety
☐ dehydration
☐ emaciation
☐ insomnia
☐ wasting
☐ asthma
☐ loss of voice
☐ hoarseness
☐ tuberculosis
☐ hiccups
☐ dry cough
☐ senility
☐ tension head-
  aches
☐ shortness of
  breath

Udana Vata

☐ sore throat
☐ cancer
☐ tonsillitis
☐ stuttering
☐ weakness
☐ dry cough
☐ fatigue
☐ earaches
☐ dry eyes
☐ lack of
  enthusiasm
☐ over-excitement
☐ speech defects

Samana Vata

☐ indigestion
☐ low energy
☐ diarrhea
☐ dehydration
☐ poor nutrition
☐ too slow food
  movement
☐ too fast food
  movement

Apana Vata

☐ constipation
☐ diarrhea
☐ diabetes
☐ dysmenorrhea
☐ stillbirth
☐ difficult birth
☐ low back pain
☐ menstrual
  disorders
☐ sexual
  dysfunction

Vyana Vata

☐ joint-cracking
☐ nervousness
☐ arthritis
☐ frequent blinking
☐ heart irregularity
☐ poor circulation
☐ difficult body
  movement

PITTA

Pachaka Pitta

☐ulcers   ☐addictions
☐indigestion   ☐cravings
☐heartburn

Ranjaka Pitta

☐anger   ☐skin
☐liver disease   inflammations
☐hostility   ☐blood disorders
☐jaundice   ☐low blood
☐anemia   pressure

Sadhaka Pitta

☐heart attack   ☐emotional
☐indecision   disturbance

Alochaka Pitta

☐eye diseases   ☐visual problems
☐anger   ☐red, irritated eyes

Bhrajaka Pitta

☐acne   ☐skin cancer
☐inflammation   ☐rashes
☐poor memory   ☐all skin disorders
☐boils

KAPHA

Bodhaka Kapha

☐obesity ☐loss of taste
☐diabetes ☐food sensitivity
☐congestion

Avalambaka Kapha

☐asthma ☐stiffness
☐back pains ☐chest
☐lethargy   congestion

Kledaka Kapha

☐slow digestion ☐excess mucous
☐fullness   in stomach

Slesaka Kapha

☐loose joints ☐slow, painful
☐swelling   movements
☐stiffness

Tarpaka Kapha

☐headaches ☐irritability
☐loss of smell ☐sinus irritation

CHAPTER FIVE

LIFESTYLE AND DIET

GENERAL GUIDANCE FOR BALANCING THE DOSHAS

The remainder of this book is primarily concerned with the use of essential oils in balancing the doshas. Please remember, essential oils are only an adjunct to dosha balancing; lifestyle and diet are more important. Fortunately, essential oils can help create changes in lifestyle and can be added to the diet. This chapter is intended as a quick reference guide to assist in your day to day living.

Reducing Vata

General Information: Consume warm foods and drinks, unctuous (oily) food, foods with predominately sweet, sour and salty tastes. Oil your body every day with sesame and essential oils. It is best not to eat alone. Best colors for meditation are yellow, orange, red. Avoid dark colors. Best stones are jade, peridot. Best metal is gold. Avoid cold wind, dampness, excess travel, television, radio, movies, excess talking and thinking. Practice yoga that is calming and grounding. Exercise should be non-vigorous and non-ex-haustive, such as tai chi, walking or swimming. Use bulk and tonic laxatives like flax seed and psyllium. Avoid diet and fasting, dry foods, cold foods and drinks, and foods having predominantly pungent, bitter or astringent tastes. Meals should be small but frequent. It is important to go to bed before 10 p.m. If prone to insomnia, drink teas at night that are calming and soothing. Vata types do better in warm, moist climates. When they live in a cold climate, it is important to protect the head, neck and chest, and keep warm. Use routines to ground, calm and stabilize your life.

Reducing Pitta

General Information: Cool foods and drinks are best; foods with predominately sweet, bitter and astringent tastes. Avoid food with pungent, sour and salty tastes. Have flowers around the house. Bathe in moonlight. Take walks in the cool air. At night, massage your scalp with coconut oil. Competitive team sports, which promote cooperation, are ideal; also activities like hiking, which are vigorous and not ego-producing. The best stones, to be carried on the right side of the body, are sapphire, aquamarine, azurite. Take flower baths. Do regular liver flushes: juice of 1 lemon, 1 tbl. olive oil, 1 small diced apple or other fruit, blend and drink instead of breakfast (Vata and Kapha may add ginger, garlic and cayenne). Follow diet and avoid restricted foods whenever possible. For meditation colors, use blue and green. Best metal to use on the body is silver. Avoid excessive sauna, hot tub or sunbathing. Seek out what gives you joy.

Reducing Kapha

General Information: Fast once a week for twenty-four hours. Foods with pungent, bitter and astringent tastes are best. Avoid or reduce sweet, sour and salty foods. No breakfast before 10 a.m., light meal in the evening. Frequent physical and mental exercise; sexual intercourse. Minimum sleep. Best colors are yellow, brown and red. Best stones are yellow topaz, coral and diamond. Best metals to use on the body are copper or iron. Take regular baths and saunas to promote sweating.

DIETS FOR REDUCING IMBALANCE

Diet for Reducing Vata Imbalance

	YES		AVOID/REDUCE	
GRAINS	(cooked well)		barley	granola
	basmati rice	oats	buckwheat	millet
	brown rice	wheat	corn	no dry cereals
FRUITS	avocado	mango	apple	melon
	banana	melons	cranberry	pear
	cantaloupe	papaya	dried fruits	pomegranate
	cherries	peaches		
	coconut	persimmons		
	fresh figs	sweet berries		
	grapes	sweet fruits		
	grapefruit	sweet orange		
	lemon	sweet		
	lime	pineapple		
	mandarin	sweet plums		
VEGETABLES	well-cooked vegetables (with butter, lemon)		bean sprouts	eggplant
	beets	sweet potato	broccoli	green beans
	carrots	tomatoes	brussels sprouts	lettuce
	cucumber	turnips	cabbage	peas
	Jerusalem artichokes	winter squash	cauliflower	potato
	mushrooms	yams	celery	raw vegetables
	okra	kale	cilantro	spinach
	pickled vegetables	zucchini	corn, fresh	
ANIMAL FOODS (for non-vegetarians)	chicken	sea food	beef	rabbit
	lamb	turkey	pheasant	
	pork			

Diet for Reducing Vata Imbalance
(continued)

	YES		AVOID/REDUCE	
DAIRY	all dairy products, especially fermented like yogurt, buttermilk and keifer			
BEANS	made into a paste or dahl: chick peas (humus), mung beans, pink lentils		all beans should be avoided except for pulses (dahl), green beans and tofu	
OILS	all oils, but best sesame oil and ghee, mayonnaise		corn oil	mustard oil
SPICES	allspice anise asafoetida basil bay black pepper (small amts.) caraway cardamon cinnamon	clove coriander cumin fennel garlic ginger onion salt tarragon thyme	cayenne chili juniperberry mustard	nutmeg peppermint sage turmeric
NUTS AND SEEDS	all nuts		peanuts-dry roasted	
SWEETENERS	sugar cane products	molasses rice syrup	raw honey	carob
BEVERAGES	hot herbal teas warm rice milk	1 small glass wine (no sulfites) with meals	cold drinks coffee	black tea all other alcohols

Diet for Reducing Pitta Imbalance

	YES		AVOID/REDUCE	

GRAINS	barley
	buckwheat
	oat
	soda breads &
	  pancakes
		wheat, rye
		white rice
		  (basmati)
		corn - blue
			brown rice
			corn - yellow
				millets
				yeasted
				  breads

FRUITS	coconut cherries grapes mango melons pear	pomegranate sweet fruits sweet oranges sweet pineapple sweet plums	avocado grapefruit lemon juice limes olives	papaya peaches persimmon sour oranges sour pineapple
VEGETABLES	asparagus broccoli brussels sprouts cabbage cauliflower celery cucumber green beans mushrooms	okra peas potato pumpkin steamed onions (sweet) sweet potato turnips zucchini	beets carrots chard chilies eggplant garlic hot peppers mustard greens	onion parsley pickles purple peppers radish spinach tomato white onions

DAIRY	butter
	cottage cheese
	cream cheese
	ghee
		milk
		rice dream
		soybean ice
		  cream
			cheese
			cultured
			  buttermilk
			kefir
				salty cheeses
				sour cream
				yogurt

BEANS	most beans, especially mung, tofu, aduki, black, chickpeas, lima, soybeans, fava		lentils, especially red	

Diet for Reducing Pitta Imbalance
(continued)

	YES		AVOID/REDUCE	
SPICES	cardamon	fennel	cayenne	nutmeg
	cilantro	lemongrass	celery seeds	pepper
	cinnamon	lemon skin	clove	oregano
	coriander	lotus seeds	fenugreek	rosemary
	cumin	mint	ginger	sage, salt
	dill	turmeric	mustard seed	all other spices
NUTS AND SEEDS	best if sprouted	lotus seed	almonds	pine nuts
		sunflower	cashews	pumpkin
	coconut	(best not in summer)	peanuts	sesame seeds
SWEETENERS	maple syrup	stivia	in moderation	
	rice syrup	barley	honey	white sugar
			molasses	
BEVERAGES	cold drinks	soy milk	alcohol	hot drinks
			coffee, tea	
BEST TO AVOID/ REDUCE	fermented products			
	meat			
	salt			
	tobacco			

Diet for Reducing Kapha Imbalance

	YES		AVOID/REDUCE	
GRAINS	basmati rice buckwheat corn	rye roasted grains	barley brown rice oats	wheat white rice millet
FRUITS	apple cranberry dried fruit kiwi pear	persimmon pomegranate raisins strawberry	banana coconut dates figs grapes melons	orange papaya pineapple prunes sweet fruits
VEGETABLES	artichokes asparagus beets bitter melon bok choy broccoli cabbage carrots cauliflower celery chili eggplant green pepper	green salads hot pepper leafy greens lettuce mushrooms mustard greens onions potatoes radish spinach sprouts squash swiss chard	cucumber okra sweet potatoes tomatoes	zucchini sweet and juicy vegetables
DAIRY	goat milk ghee	small amt. unsalted buttermilk	most dairy	
BEANS	all beans: aduki, fava, kidney, lentils, lima		tofu in ex- treme Kapha	chickpeas humus

Diet for Reducing Kapha Imbalance
(continued)

	YES	AVOID/REDUCE
OILS	(small amounts) almond mustard canola soy corn sunflower	all others
SWEETENERS	small amount only, raw, uncooked honey	all other sweeteners
NUTS AND SEEDS	best if pumpkin seed sprouted sunflower flax seed	peanuts all others
ANIMAL FOODS (for non-vegetarians)	fresh water fish turkey rabbit (dark meat) venison	beef seafood chicken fat, no fried or lamb, pork greasy food
SPICES	all spices, especially garlic and ginger	pickles vinegar salt
BEVERAGES	almond milk ginger tea coffee (1 cup/ old wine, 1 sm. day) glass w/meals cranberry juice tea	ice cold drinks

CHAPTER SIX

TOXINS AND DISEASE

Metabolism is the ingestion and burning up (chemically) of raw materials to energize the body. All combustion, even in the body, produces waste residues that have natural channels of elimination. Ayurveda calls these waste products *ama*. The residues of human metabolism exit the body via the lungs, the skin, the liver and colon, and the kidneys. In addition to our normal metabolic waste products, in the industrial age we have all types of toxic residues such as heavy metals, pesticides, herbicides, food additives, and food preservatives. All of these can enter into our metabolism via our food, water, and air supply. Science calls these accumulated residues "toxic load."

Very often our lifestyles don't promote the natural elimination of all of these residues. Harvey Diamond, in his book *Fit For Life*, says that the body's natural time period for elimination begins at night and extends until the first meal of the day. Modern eating practices of late meals, midnight snacks and early breakfasts cut down on this time of elimination. He recommends fruits and light foods in the morning until noon to extend that eliminative period. This is especially appropriate for a person who is toxic or overweight.

Ayurveda says that a diminishing of digestive fire is often a first step in the buildup of toxins. Like a low flame, it is unable to completely burn the fuel under which it is placed, and leaves a trail of thick smoke. The residues of incomplete digestion are transported by Vata to inherited weak areas in the body, blocking important channels and vessels.

Ayurveda teaches that if we have no weaknesses, the doshas can increase to any level with no ill effect. But the more weaknesses we have, the more critical it is to maintain our balance. If the excess doshas and ama (waste products) are transported to the heart, we have coronary heart disease. If they are transported to the joints, the doctors tell us we have arthritis. Wherever they travel, there is disease.

SIX STAGES OF DISEASE

There are six progressive stages of disease. Disease does not just appear; there is no such thing as a "sudden heart attack." Years of imbalance and neglect create that experience.

The first stage of disease is called **accumulation** and is begun when there is an imbalance in the doshas and a buildup in the specific areas of the body. This may occur because of inappropriate diet, lifestyle, thoughts or feelings.

The second stage, **aggravation**, is a sign that the dosha has begun to overflow like a bucket of water under a dripping faucet.

The third stage, **dissemination**, is the excess dosha moving throughout the body. During this stage, there can be a whole range of symptoms occurring in different parts of the body at different times—vague symptoms that are rather hard for the patient or a doctor to pin down.

The fourth stage is known as **relocation**. This is the stage where the imbalanced dosha has settled into one specific site and begun to cause more serious symptoms.

The fifth stage is **manifestation**, where the excess dosha has settled down and can now be identified as a specific disease.

The last stage is known as **disruption**, because the disease manifests, disrupting the health of the individual. It is at this stage that a medical physician can recognize definitively what is wrong, and give the disease a name.

PROGRESSION THROUGH THE SIX STAGES OF DISEASE

1. Accumulation

An individual may begin by eating a diet which is too light and too dry during a cold and dry season, without adequate protection from dry, cold wind. This upsets the metabolism, blood flow, mental state and digestion. Vata begins to accumulate in the colon, causing gas, constipation, and inability to sleep.

2. Aggravation

Symptoms increase, including abdominal pains and spasms, increased gas and increased constipation.

3. Dissemination

Symptoms such as dry skin, joint stiffness, headaches and painful bowel movements begin to occur.

4. Relocation

The joint pain becomes the most prominent of symptoms.

5. Manifestation

The dis-ease can now be identified as arthritis.

6. Disruption

The specific manifestations of Vata arthritis, coldness, stiffness, dryness and the severe pain, will be evident.

The earlier an imbalance in the doshas is discovered, and the earlier treatment commences, the easier it is to remedy imbalance. In the earlier stages, simple removal of the toxins, residues and excess doshas will return the body to balance and health. In the later stages, tissue has been damaged, and treatment will take longer. Once the ama is removed, the body can rebuild the damaged tissue, but this can require up to a year of being in balance.

Pancha karma is a seasonal Ayurvedic cleansing therapy that encourages all the elimination systems. In addition to Pancha karma, in the latter stages of disease, Rasayana, or rejuvenation therapy, will be necessary to encourage the body to rebuild the damaged tissue.

In Section II, the reader will learn how essential oils can assist body metabolism, promote ama removal, and help balance the doshas.

SECTION II

AROMATHERAPY
and
ESSENTIAL OILS

Bryan: I first became aware of essential oils when Light and I owned a holistic clinic in Sacramento, California. I was the "doctor" and she was in charge of all the massage therapists. I noticed that she and the massage therapists were running around with these little bottles of oils—mixing them together, creating special formulations for different patients. And it didn't seem very scientific to me. While I vaguely knew that they were using lavender, sandalwood and other scents, I didn't know where they came from, what they could do, or how much they cost. I should have become suspicious when my wife asked me if she could purchase an ounce of rose oil and split it with two other friends, because she rarely asks my permission for anything. I said yes, not thinking. Several days later she proudly showed me her portion of the rose oil, and mentioned the price, $150. I hit the ceiling—in a red-eyed, tunnel-vision rage. "How in the world could you possibly spend $150 for something I could pour in the palm of my hand?" With her most pure, instinctual reflex, she opened the bottle and thrust it under my nose, and said simply, "smell." I felt my anger diminish exponentially with each breath. "My God," I said, "I can't believe how wonderful that smells and how good I feel at this moment." From then on I began to pay attention to all those little bottles.

CHAPTER SEVEN

ESSENTIAL OILS THROUGH TIME

EARLY USE OF AROMATICS

Early humans lived a natural and intimate experience with nature. All of their senses were acutely attuned to any change in the external environment. Smell, being ten thousand times more sensitive than taste, was an extremely important sense for survival, signaling the presence of dangerous animals and enemies, assisting in the location of food, even signaling the availability of a member of the opposite sex. Coming straight from the womb, a baby is able to differentiate its mother from every other female and immediately find its important first nourishment—the breast—all through the sense of smell.

On the walls of the caves of Lascaux, France, are pictures from 18000 BC, showing illustrations of medicinal plants. The body of an ice-age man was found thawing in a glacier on the border between Austria and Italy; the oldest person to appear on the cover of *Time*, he is thought to have been a Shaman, because bundles of herbs were found in a pouch at his side.

Early man associated bad smells with disfavor of the gods, illness and disease. A healthy person had a clean and fresh odor. Early man observed sick animals feeding on special herbs, and saw them recover their health; in this way they accumulated plant wisdom, the beginnings of herbology. They discovered that herbs and spices helped to preserve food, aided in digestion, and enhanced taste. When early man accidentally spilled some herbs on a fire, he found the smoke to be pleasing and wholesome, and began to burn resin and dried herbs for purification rituals. Herbs and aromatics became one of the few things important enough to carry, preserve and maintain. Primitive man saw in every plant a gift from the creator, a secret to be revealed, a plant ally to be cherished, a way of coming back into health and favor of the gods. When men settled into a fertile river valley and decided to plant seeds into the ground and raise domestic animals, they brought with them the sacred herbs that had become their medicine.

THE EGYPTIANS

The Egyptians achieved such a high level of civilization that the secrets of the pyramids and their construction have yet to be fully explained. Papyrus records from 4500 BC tell of the use of balsam, perfumed oils, scented barks and resins and the production of aromatic vinegars, wines and beer. The specific formulations were blended by the priests, who interpreted the will of the Gods for the people, and were also physicians. They recorded recipes for illness, for restoring youthfulness, for hay fever, and for contraception.

We know now that Egyptian temples were laboratories for the high priest. Valued herbs and flowers were imported from as far away as Somalia, Malaysia, India and China: seeds such as caraway and anise, roots such as angelica and blue orchid, barks such as

An Egyptian Recipe for Contraception

Acacia, coloquinte, dates and honey, blended together and placed in the vagina, where natural bacteria caused fermentation, the creation of lactic acid, and spermicidal action.

cedarwood and cypress, and resins such as frankincense and myrrh. The priests used hundreds of thousands of pounds of plants to make scented oils to be burned in the temples. The statues of the gods were covered with special oils for each god and goddess (artemisia for Isis, marjoram for Osiris). The Egyptian vocabulary for smell was extraordinarily extensive, a linguistic indicator of the importance of smell in the culture. They had perfumes for different occasions—morning, evening, meditation, love, war. The Pharaohs and their family members had signature perfumes composed like music especially for

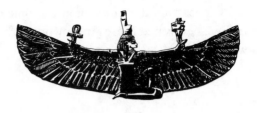

Isis

them. Queen Hatshepsut, the only female Pharaoh (1490-1468 BC), promoted the development of perfumes and the bold eye makeup that is associated with the Egyptians.

The Egyptians believed that the physical body was important in the afterlife and they discovered that aromatics and essential oils had preservative effects. The art of embalming developed. Each embalmer developed his secret formula, which was fiercely guarded. The embalming process involved withdrawing the brain and removing the viscera, which were then stored in different pots in a solution of sodium carbonate. The body was bathed with essential oils and soaked in aromatic resins. After three months, the body was wrapped in gauze impregnated with resin, cedarwood oil and myrrh. For royalty, the entire process took as much as six months, while on a common man, it might take only a few hours. So successful was the process that fragments of intestine three thousand years old, when examined under a microscope, were found to be completely intact. The wrappings of the early discovered mummies were transported back to England and France soaked in alcohol, and the strained solution was sold as a medicine to increase resistance to disease.

Ordinary Egyptians used aromatics extensively in cooking. They used anise, coriander, and caraway added to their millet and barley bread to increase digestibility. Mint, marjoram and parsley were widely used as flavorings in food. Onion was often substituted for meat, and a bulb was found beside every mummy. The inscription on the pyramid of Cheops (4500 BC) states, "Every morning each slave will be provided a clove of garlic by his master for health and strength during construction."

An early deodorant was developed by the Egyptians; aromatics molded into a wax cone would melt during the heat of the day and release fragrant smells.

Cleopatra, ruler of Egypt at the time of the Roman expansion, was said to have bewitched Marc Antony not with her looks, but through her artistry with perfume.

PARALLEL DEVELOPMENT - OTHER CULTURES

Civilizations in Mesopotamia, India and China traded not only herbal and aromatic products, but information on how to use them. A clay distillation apparatus was discovered in Persia that dates back to 2500 BC. Clay tablets revealed that, in Babylon, 57,000 pounds of frankincense was burned every year.

In the civilization of Assyria, 60 tons of frankincense were used every year in the annual feast of the god Baal. In the kingdom of Israel, at the funeral of Herod, 5,000 slaves preceded the king's body, carrying urns of burning frankincense.

In India, Ayurveda had embraced herbs and aromatics as an important part of the philosophy of healing, using fresh herbs, dried herbs as tea, or dried or fresh herbs compounded into a powder and often formed into hand-rolled pills, using fresh plant juices. An early form of essential oil extraction involved pounding and grinding the fresh or dried herb, and subsequent squeezing or expressing of the essential oil.

The art of steam distillation, using ceramic or pottery stills, was perfected three to four thousand years ago and is still in use today. Trade and wars brought many new herbs to India from the Far East, the Middle East, Egypt and Africa. Arab conquests in the Indian subcontinent a thousand years ago brought huge changes in the use of essential oils. The Arabs' distillation expertise allowed for the making of attars, using a co-distillation method where a very light volatile essential

---

The Discovery of Rose Oil

A Raj of India held a huge celebration for the marriage of his daughter. As part of the preparation for the festivities, he ordered the moat around the castle to be filled with rose petals. After the celebration was over, people noticed a film on the water that, when tasted or smelled, contained the essence of rose. Thus began the production of rose essential oil which continues to be important in Bulgaria, Romania, Turkey and India.

---

component, such as jasmine, can be distilled with a very heavy essential oil component like sandalwood, and the heavier component traps the light flowery component. Essential oil production continues to be an important industry in many small villages where the distillation apparatus designs have not changed for 3,000 years.

Greek and Roman Use of Aromatherapy

The Greeks, then the Romans, borrowed heavily from the Egyptians and contact with the Indian culture in their use of aromatherapeutics, perfumes, scented oils and in their understanding of herbal medicine. Perfuming the body was an important aspect of life; essential oil massage was a therapeutic regimen recommended by Hippocrates to be performed daily. It is said that the Roman emperor Nero commanded that an entire year's production of frankincense be burned at the funeral of his wife, Sabina Poppae. An entire fleet of ships was used solely to transport frankincense from Arabia to Rome.

The Latin meaning of the word perfuma means "by smoke" and was originally applied to the burning of incense. The Greeks and Romans marketed the first commercial perfume, a reproduction of the Egyptian recipe named kyphi, dating from 1500 BC. Though it was said to contain sixteen herbs, the translation contained only twelve.

(Partial) Recipe for Kyphi (the worlds' first perfume)

calamus, cassia, cinnamon, cyperus, frankincense, hina, juniper, mastic, myrrh, saffron, spikenard, terebinth

CHRISTIAN EUROPE

With the downfall of the Roman Empire, Europe descended into the dark ages. Many important facets of healing with aromatics was lost to this part of the world, particularly the secret of the distillation process. All literary knowledge was confined to the monasteries, as was herbal knowledge. The monks became not only the interpreters of God's will, but also the dispensers of His healing as they used the medicinals from their herbal gardens and dispensed medication in the form of herbal teas, herbal infused oils, medicated beers, medicated wines, brandies, and herbal tinctures.

During the middle ages, the plague (black death) was most feared, and some people realized that aromatic substances might be a defense against the contagion. It was well documented that herbalists and perfumers were virtually immune. A particularly bold band of thieves was able to rob the houses of the dead with impunity because the thieves drank a vinegar tincture soaked with aromatic herbs and spices, thus making them immune to contagion when entering the houses of the afflicted. In time the authorities extracted this information from the thieves (in return for a lighter sentence), and the formula became available and used by many. During times of plague, fumigation by burning aromatic woods such as pine, cedar and cypress was employed both inside the home and in the open street.

The modern rediscovery of essential oils is credited to the Arabian physician and philosopher Avicenna (1000 AD). The Arabs taught chemistry, the healing use of plants, and distillation methods at their universities, including the universities in Spain. During the Holy Crusades and the conquest of Spain, Arab allies shared the secrets of distillation. Information on this lost process was carried back to Europe. By 1200 AD, 47 different essential oils were being distilled in Germany. Early production centered around the well-known and time-honored aromatic herbs, spices and resins from the Far East, the Middle East and Africa. Gradually, the distillation of northern herbs increased, and therapeutic knowledge about mint, rosemary, chamomile and other temperate herbs became widespread. By the 1800s, sanitation practices had reduced the occurrence of contagious disease in the European cities, also reducing the need for herbs.

MODERN HISTORY

Up until the early 1900s, essential oils were the strongest medicine available. A shift began with the development of powerful coal tar derivatives and preparations. This was the beginning of pharmacology and allopathic medicine.

The modern father of aromatherapy is considered to be Dr. Rene-Maurice Gattefosse. He was a French chemist who worked in his family's perfume laboratory. One day when he suffered a severe burn from an explosion in the lab, he quickly thrust his injured hand into a container of lavender oil and was amazed to notice the immediate decrease in pain, and subsequently observed rapid healing with no scarring. So impressed was he by this experience that he dedicated the rest of his life to researching and discovering the therapeutic properties of essential oils on the most scientific basis. He first coined the word "aromatherapy" and published a book by that name in 1937.

A French medical doctor, Dr. Jean Valnet, was greatly influenced by Gattafosse's work. During the second World War, he experienced success treating war injuries with antiseptic essential oil solutions. In 1964, he published a book called *Aromatherapy Treatment of Illnesses by the Essence of Plants*, and he is responsible for training over 1,000 French physicians currently using essential oils in their practice. Essential oils have been accepted as valid therapy in France, and a prescription for essential oils can be filled at the local pharmacy and paid for by insurance.

Numerous experiments have proven the antiseptic qualities of essential oils (i.e., thyme is eight times more powerful than phenol). Russian researchers have verified the stimulation of liver digestive processes by rose oil. Italian researchers have verified the psychological effects of essential oil. The anti-viral and anti-fungal properties create the most exciting application possibilities as medicine has little to offer for the treatment of virus.

One of Dr. Valnet's students, Margarite Mallory, further developed the modern use of essential oils in massage therapy and skin care in England.

In this country, the American Aromatherapy Association was founded in 1987 by Victoria Edwards, Kurt Schnaubelt and Marcelle Lavabre. They and Robert Tisserand are largely responsible for the spread of aromatherapy in the United States.

The use of aromatherapy continues to increase in the U.S. as people become aware of the limitations of modern medicine, the importance of self care, and the high potency of essential oils.

CHAPTER EIGHT

WHAT ARE ESSENTIAL OILS?

*E*ssential oils are the aromatic or volatile constituents found in plants. They contain the most active physiological properties. Some experts say they contain the life force of the plant. Chemically, essential oils are made up of alcohols, aldehydes, ketones, phenols, terpenes, sesquiterpenes, ethers and esters, which we shall talk about later in detail. In the living plant, these essential oil components are used as hormones for growth and reproduction, plant pheromones for smells which will attract pollinating insects, defense mechanisms protecting the plant from predators (herbivores and insects), and also protection against bacterial, viral, or fungal invasion. Some plants have very high concentrations of essential oils, which they have developed for protection. We call them herbs, and have used them for thousands of years to add to our own body's arsenals of defense.

Essential oils can be derived from all parts of the plant. The flowers produce essential oils that often have sedating, narcotic or relaxing effects on the body. The resins, woods, barks and exudates produce heating essential oils that actively move fluids in the body. The leaves often have healing and cooling properties coming from the green color of chlorophyll (very closely related to our hemoglobin structure). The roots contain many of the earth properties of the plants and can be very grounding. The fruits produce essential oils that are very expanding, opening and stimulating. We can use these essential oil properties to alter our dosha imbalances.

PRODUCTION METHODS

There are many methods to extract the aromatic qualities from plants. Teas, tinctures, decoctions, infused oils, herbal beers, and wines all extract and concentrate the volatile components of the plants—but these are not essential oils. Essential oils are much more concentrated, and are produced by steam distillation, cold pressing, CO_2 hyperbaric extraction, and solvent extraction. Each method has its advantages and disadvantages and produces a different quality of oil.

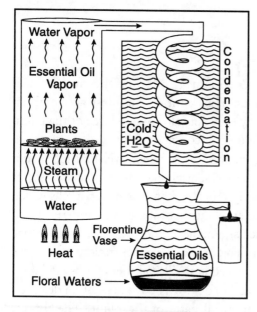

Steam Distillation

Steam distillation is the most common method of essential oil extraction.

Distillation uses the extraction abilities of steam, and sometimes pressure, to pull the aromatic qualities from the plant material. The chosen plant material is placed on screens over boiling water, or super-heated steam from another source is piped through the plant material. As the steam passes through the plant material, the volatile components are lifted, condensed in a cooling coil, and precipitate out as a combination of distilled water and volatile components. The mixture is collected in a florentine vase (which has an hourglass shape) and in most cases the distilled water is heavier and sinks to the bottom, while the essential oils, being lighter, rise to the top, at which point a valve can be opened and the essential oils drained off.

There are very primitive methods of steam distillation that use very low heat and may take as long as a month to distill one batch of essential oils. The advantage in "slow" distillation is that the long time (and patience) allows some of the larger molecules to be gently coaxed out, and can produce an essence which has a wider range of smells. More modern methods of distillation may use higher temperatures to very quickly extract essential oils, sometimes in a matter of minutes. This can produce oils quickly, cheaply and efficiently; however, the bouquet, or range of smells, is somewhat restricted by this method, and involves a loss in some of the possible therapeutic qualities.

Cold pressing is the second most common method of essential oil production and is most useful in the processing of citrus rinds such as lemon, orange, grapefruit, tangerine, bergamot and mandarin. The rinds, or in some cases the whole fruit, are chopped or ground, and pressed to extract the essential oil components that are found in the skin of the fruit. In early days, and in some places in the world today, the rinds of these fruits were squeezed into sponges. Take a piece of citrus rind, fold it, skin out, and notice the spray of essential oils (watch your eyes). Do this into a candle flame and witness the flash of blue as the volatiles ignite.

Cold pressing produces a combination of essential oils and watery components which can be allowed to separate and the essential components collected. The mechanical nature of this process produces essential oils which are not as pure, and tend to oxidize or lose their potency if left unrefrigerated for more than two years. Steam-distilled essential oil, on the other hand, will grow richer in smell over the years and in some cases have unlimited shelf life.

The **CO2 hyperbaric production** method utilizes as much as 22 atmospheres of pressure in the presence of pure CO_2 gas (the same pressure found at ocean depths of 660 feet). At high pressure the CO_2 becomes liquid and has the ability to extract the essential oil components from the plant material. This liquid is drained off and allowed to depressurize, at which point the CO_2 becomes a harmless gas. What's left in the bottom of the chamber is pure essential oil. This method is especially useful in some of the lighter fragrances such as tuberose or jasmine where the flowers have light, easily lost aromatic components. The cost of the compression equipment is great and oils produced are more expensive than steam distilled.

The **solvent extraction method** is also useful with light aromatic flowers. The flowers are collected and a solvent such as hexane or ether poured over them. The solvents are evaporated using a vacuum, and what's left is a very thick, sticky residue known as a "concrete." The concrete can be dissolved in alcohol, the alcohol pulled off, and the remaining essential oil is known as an "absolute." Perfumers like this method because it doesn't involve heat, pressure, or mechanical pressing which can change the odor of the flowers. Perfumers maintain that absolutes are more true to the original smell of the flower than oils produced using any other method of production. Aromatherapists, however, know that a small amount of the petroleum solvent always remains and can be harmful to the human immune system, causing reactions in sensitive people. In aromatherapy, it is the method least preferred, and oils produced in this manner are never used internally.

CARE AND SELECTION OF ESSENTIAL OILS

Essential oils are light-sensitive and should be stored in tightly capped amber or colored bottles away from extremes of heat or cold. Anything being sold in a clear bottle is most likely not an essential oil. Clear glass, at the very least, can indicate distribution by people unfamiliar with essential oils. Essential oils should be labeled with the botanical name of the extracted plant and information should be available about the method used to produce them. Essential oils vary greatly in price due to production variables. It can take up to 2,000 pounds of rose petals to produce one pound of rose essential oil through distillation. Lavender flowers can produce essential oils at a ratio of 50 to 1; 25 pounds of citrus rind make one pound of expressed citrus oils. Due to the variables of labor, rainfall, farming costs, extraction methods, and demand on the world market, rose oil can sell for $400 or more for one ounce and orange for as little as $3. If you see different essential oils selling for the same price, it is probable that these oils are diluted with vegetable oil to create this pricing structure. Beware of fragrances usually sold in clear glass. These are not essential oils, but are chemical compositions made in a laboratory to produce a smell which is a copy of nature. There is no such essential oil as watermelon, bubble gum or piña colada. Perfumes may contain essential oil components—the finer perfumes invariably do—but they also contain petroleum products (fragrance) and alcohol to increase their diffusability (movement into the air).

CHAPTER NINE

ESSENTIAL OILS AND THE BODY INTERFACE

HOW AND WHY ESSENTIAL OILS AFFECT THE BODY

The routes through which essential oils react with the body and its metabolism are called pathways. In the first phase, essential oils penetrate the epithelial tissues; these include the skin, nasal passages, bronchioles, lungs and gastro-intestinal tract.

Once absorbed into the surface layer, essential oils quickly penetrate into the lymphatic and blood capillary systems, entering into the general circulation. This is true for the other epithelial tissues of the body, including sinuses and lungs. The essential oils in the lymph circulatory system can be carried directly to the liver or fed into the blood stream. As the oils circulate with the blood, body tissues and organs may choose any portion of the essential oil that it wishes to utilize in its metabolic processes, or simply receive the stimulation, sedation, or beneficial property of the oil as it passes through. It is important to remember that nothing stays in the body very long (consider the hundreds of pounds of food and drink that we consume on a monthly basis). Essential oils, because of their volatile nature, usually leave the body within 48 hours.

MODE OF ENTRY	CIRCULATION	ORGANS & TISSUES	Picked up from Circulation	EXCRETION
Liquid - Skin GI Tract	Capillaries Blood & Lymph Generalized Circulation to Whole Body	Oils Circulating in the Body Affect Muscle, Fat, Joints, Organs All Tissues		Skin - Sebaceous Glands
				Lungs - Vapor
Vapor - Sinus Lung				Kidneys - Urine
				Liver - Bile - GI Tract Feces
Nerve Impulse Smell	Olfactory Nerve	Limbic System Reptilian Brain	Triggers Memories Emotions Desires Appetites	Neuropeptides, Hormones & Neurotransmitter Release

The essential oils will have a strong effect on these primary contact tissues.

The third stage of the pathways involves the elimination process. Some components of essential oils are picked up by the surface of the lungs and are outgassed as a vapor. Eucalyptol (an alcohol in eucalyptus oil) is transported to the lung surfaces by the blood stream and calms the mucous membranes as it exits. Others, such as the terpenes in juniperberry oil, are filtered out by the kidneys, and have a stimulating effect on the renal tissue, ureters, bladder and urethra as they exit. Some components of the essential oils are extracted by the liver, held briefly in the gall bladder, and dumped into the GI tract, having profound affects on these organ systems as they pass through. Rose oil stimulates bile production as it is processed by the liver. Some constituents tend to migrate toward the skin, where they will exit via the sebaceous glands and become part of the protective acid mantle (coating). Components of yarrow increase perspiration as they are excreted. Soap is damaging to the skin because its alkalinity removes the acid mantle. People who understand cosmetics use PH balanced products that won't strip and expose the skin to dryness and infection. The essential oils that move through this pathway are added to our protective layer.

The most important pathway, in terms of its profound effect on the body, is through the sense of smell. When we smell essential oils, the vapor stimulates small hair-like extensions of our olfactory nerve. The olfactory nerve is the only nerve in the body that directly contacts the external environment and goes all the way to the brain. All of our other senses (touch, hearing, sight, and taste) involve several nerves and synaptic junctions before the impulses reach the brain. The olfactory nerve stimulates the most primitive part of the brain known as the limbic system, also called the saurian or reptilian brain. This is important in the processing of and reaction to emotions, desires, appetites and memories. This direct connection is why essential oils can have such profound and immediate effects on a very deep aspect of our beingness. Research indicates that very small (almost homeopathic) quantities create this stimulation. Larger doses do not increase the response appreciably.

Flower Essence Creates a Night of Passion

At a trade show in Anaheim, California, we gave out samples of champa, a flower blend from India, which is exotic, sweet and euphoric. One of the buyers returned excitedly the next day requesting more. She explained that she had tried the champa on herself, and upon returning home, her husband was all over her, asking about her day, what she had seen, touching her and gazing intently into her eyes; all very uncharacteristic behavior. He carried her to the bedroom and they experienced a passion like never before. She knew it had to be the champa and had to have more.

CHAPTER TEN

AYURVEDIC CHEMISTRY

WESTERN AROMATHERAPY

Traditional Western use of both herbs and aromatics is to classify them and use them according to general therapeutic properties. In this system, a symptom such as indigestion is often matched with categories of herbs that are known to help it, in this case a classification known as carminatives. This system of working symptomatically with herbs and oils is the end result of thousands of years of animal observation and human experimentation. The good thing about this system is that it does provide information on the properties of the various herbs. Its drawback is that there are situations where an herb may be selected that is appropriate for the symptom, but not appropriate for the patient, and may produce an ill effect. An example might be a Pitta (fire) person searching an herbal book for help with indigestion, and finding carminatives with a choice of coriander or oregano, among others. Ayurveda would pick a carminative that was cooling, such as coriander; oregano, as a heating carminative, would aggravate a Pitta's condition. Ayurveda makes the distinction in the energetics of each herb and essential oil; not only the symptoms they treat, but also whether they're warming or cooling, drying or moisturizing. With these variables Ayurveda is able to take into consideration which essential oils would be best for Vata, Pitta, or Kapha types, or specific subdosha conditions.

General Therapeutic Properties

The following is a list of general therapeutic properties and their meanings. In addition to their Ayurvedic energetics, these classifications will be later applied to all listed essential oils. We acknowledge and are grateful to Dr. Vasant Lad and Dr. David Frawley for these definitions, found in *The Yoga of Herbs*.

1. **Alterative** - tending to restore normal health, cleans and purifies the blood, alters existing nutritive and excretory processes, gradually restoring normal body function.

2. **Antipyretic** - dispels heat, fire and fever (from the Greek word pyre - fire).

3. **Antispasmodic** - relieves spasms of voluntary and involuntary muscles.

4. **Aphrodisiac** - reinvigorates the body by reinvigorating the sexual organs.

5. **Astringent** - firms tissue and organs; reduces discharges and secretions.

6. **Bitter Tonic** - bitter herbs which in small amounts stimulate digestion and otherwise help regulate fire in the body.

7. **Carminative** - relieves intestinal gas pain and distention; promotes peristalsis.

8. **Diaphoretic** - causes perspiration and increased elimination through the skin.

9. **Diuretic** - promotes activity of kidney and bladder and increases urination.

10. **Emetic** - induces vomiting.

11. **Emmenagogue** - helps promote and regulate menstruation.

12. **Emollient** - smoothes, softens and protects the skin.

13. **Expectorant** - promotes discharge of phlegm and mucous from the lungs and throat.

14. **Hemostatic** - stops the flow of blood, an astringent that stops internal bleeding or hemorrhaging.

15. **Laxative** - promotes bowel movements.

16. **Nervine** - strengthens the functional activity of the nervous system; may be stimulants and sedatives.

17. **Rejuvenative** - prevents decay, postpones aging, revitalizes organs.

18. **Sedative** - calms and tranquilizes by lowering the functional activity of the organ or body part.

19. **Stimulant** - increases internal heat, dispels internal chill, strengthens metabolism and circulation.

20. **Tonic (nutritive)** - increases weight and density and nourishes the body.

21. **Vulnerary** - assists in healing of wounds by protecting against infection and stimulating cell growth.

AYURVEDIC ENERGETICS

Heating/Cooling

Ayurveda recognizes that because of their chemical makeup, all essential oils will either add heat or will have a cooling effect on the body. Essential oils can be arranged in a vertical line, with the oils that are coolest at the top, the oils that are neutral in the middle, and the oils that are warming at the bottom. All essential oils can be placed somewhere on this line, according to their properties.

Blue chamomile is a cooling oil, lavender exemplifies neutrality, and thyme is a hot essential oil. Try taking a chamomile and peppermint bath and feel the coolness when you come out. The oils in the middle range, the neutral oils such as lavender, are known as balancers, because if you're feverish, they can help to cool you down, and if you are feeling very cold and you apply lavender in a massage oil base to the body, it can help to warm you up. Lavender is an oil for all seasons. Balancers will always bring you back toward neutral, toward normal function. Experience a drop of thyme or clove rubbed into the skin on the forearm. You should notice a warmth within 15 minutes. The Oriental system of Yin and Yang corresponds directly to this, with Yin being cold and Yang being warm.

Western chemistry can fit into this arrangement, with the essential oils at the top of the chart being very electro-negative. They have extra electrons and take heat away from the body. Those essential oils at the bottom of the chart are electro-positive. They are missing electrons in their outer rings, and are eager and ready to acquire them, producing heat in the body.

The color spectrum also fits into

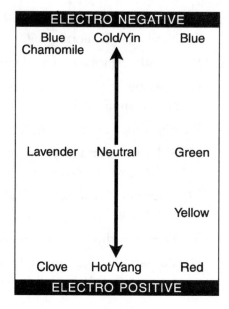

this vertical line, with red at the bottom, then orange, yellow, green in the center (neutral) and continuing to blue at the top. Many of the essential oils that are grouped along this line have the corresponding color. Oregano, thyme and savory at the bottom are very red, lemon oil has a yellow tone, the oils such as lavender, Roman chamomile and clary sage have a greenish tone, and blue chamomile at the top is a very dark blue. All the oils can therefore be classified as red-hot-yang-positive, neutral, or blue-cold-yin-negative.

Moisturizing/Drying

Ayurveda also recognizes that essential oils can be classified as wet or dry. The wet oils have high polarity and mix well with water. If you put them into a bath they disperse into, and become a part of, the water. Another name for this property is hydrophilic (water loving). Oils of low polarity don't mix with water. They will float on the surface of a bath and form a "ring" on the edge of the tub. They have affinity for and mix with vegetable oils and fats and are sometimes called lipophilic (fat loving). All of the essential oils can be arranged on a line that runs from the left (wet) to the right (dry). Some of the wet essential oils are geranium and rose, having high constituent levels of alcohol, and some of the dry, fat loving oils are the terpenes, such as

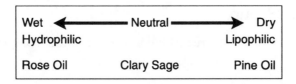

citrus oils and pine. Neutral oils again are oils such as lavender, clary sage, Roman chamomile, basil, anise, and tarragon.

It is possible, therefore, to take these two lines (one running vertically and the other running horizontally) and combine them to form a graph. By combining these two scales, each one dimensional, we can now show where the predominant energy of an oil would fall on a two-dimensional graphic. An oil that is hot and wet would fall into the lower left quadrant and correspond to an energetic description of Pitta, which, being made of water and fire elements, is hot and wet.

An essential oil that is cold and wet would appear in the upper left quadrant, and would correspond to Kapha energetics which are cold and wet. An essential oil which is cold and dry would correspond to Vata energetics and would appear in the upper right quadrant of the graph. Therefore, it is possible to arrange the essential oils on this two-dimensional graph so as to understand them in terms of the energetics of hot-cold, wet-dry, and their stimulation of Vata, Pitta, and Kapha energetics.

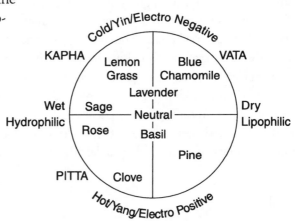

Chemical Makeup

A single essential oil can be made up of over 150 different isolated chemical constituents which work in synergy to produce various effects on the body. This can explain the different pharmacologic or therapeutic properties of a single essential oil. For instance, sage can be a diaphoretic, an expectorant, a nervine and an astringent.

Functional Groups

The various chemical constituents fall into eight functional groups.

Aldehydes

Aldehydes are known to be anti-inflammatory, calming, sedative and anti-viral. You may be familiar with form*aldehyde*, which is an industrial chemical used as a preservative. Oils containing high amounts of aldehydes would be considered Kapha-producing (being both cold and wet), and can be placed on the chart in the upper left.

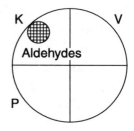

Essential oils high in aldehydes have a characteristic lemon-like smell, such as lemongrass, lemon balm, citronella, and a variety of eucalyptus called citriodora.

Cetones (also Ketones) are a class of chemicals that are wound-healing and mucolytic (eases the secretions of mucous). Their unique ability to stimulate new cell growth has been utilized in skin care. Women use *acetone* to remove nail polish (you may be chagrined to notice that essential oils can also remove the finish of your furniture if spilled). Camphor is an example of an

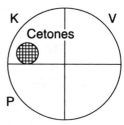

essential oil that is almost pure cetone. Other essential oils with high cetone content include rosemary, sage, eucalyptus globulus and hyssop. Cetones fall in the cold and wet category (upper left) and are Kapha-producing (cell growth). They are warmer than aldehydes but mix equally well in water.

Alcohols

Alcohols are bactericidal (kill bacteria), energizing, vitalizing, anti-viral and diuretic. The pancreas produces 32 kinds of alcohol for use in human metabolism. Some of the most beneficial molecules in essential oils are alcohols. Linalool and terpineol are two common terpene alcohols which are both ger-

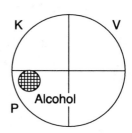

micidal and non-toxic. Essential oils which are high in alcohols include rose, petitgrain, rosewood, peppermint, myrtle, tea tree, sandalwood, patchouli and ginger. Alcohols are very wet, but only slightly heating. They fall in the left lower quadrant and stimulate Pitta (hot and wet) energetics, but not strongly.

Phenols

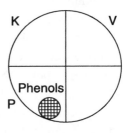

A group related to alcohols are the *phenols* which are very strongly bactericidal. They are immune stimulants, invigorating, warming, potential skin irritants and can produce slight liver toxicity if taken in high doses for extended periods of time. Pharmaceutically, phenol is used in lip balms and cough drops. Examples of oils that have high phenol content include clove, cinnamon, thyme, oregano, savory, cumin. These essential oils fall into the lower left corner of our chart and include some of the most heating of all essential oils. They produce an energetic that matches very closely the energetic of Pitta (hot and wet), and create more Pitta energy whenever they are used.

Terpenes

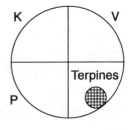

Terpenes are very stimulating, potential skin irritants and have anti-viral properties. Pine oil is used to make *terpen*tine. Oils with high amounts of terpenes include lemon, orange, bergamot, black pepper, pine oils, nutmeg and angelica. This essential oil component falls into the lower right quadrant, it is hot and dry, it does not correspond directly to any dosha energetic, but would be somewhat irritating to a Pitta condition because of the heat, and irritating to a Vata condition because of the dryness. Terpenes are some of the smallest molecules in aromatherapy, very quick to come to the nose, and very quick to evaporate.

Sesquiterpenes

Sesquiterpenes are some of the longest carbon chains found in the essential oils, very thick and tenacious, long lasting in their smell. More than two thousand sesquiterpenes have been isolated from plants, coming from the root, wood and plants of the compositae family, including such oils as blue chamomiles, immortelle, tansy, yarrow and tagetes. Properties in-

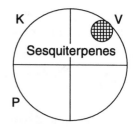

clude anti-phlogistic (moves fluids), anti-inflammatory, sedative, anti-viral, potentially anti-carcinogenic, bacteriostatic and immune stimulant. The sesquiterpenes fall in the upper right quadrant and correspond to cold and dry. Theoretically, they should produce a Vata energy, but the long-chain carbon composition and frequent combination with alcohols lessen their cooling effect. Their anti-inflammatory and immune building properties can be beneficial to all types.

Esters

Esters are chemically the most neutral of the essential oil components, being just a little above the bull's eye in the center of the chart. Esters are produced by reaction of an alcohol with an acid. They are anti-fungal, sedative, calming, spasmolytic, fungicidal, anti-inflammatory, and are known as bal-ancers or harmonizers because of their central loca-

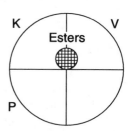

tion in the chart. They can help to normalize any energetic or condition. Essential oils containing high amounts of esters include Roman chamomile, lavender, clary sage, petitgrain, bergamot.

Lactones

Lactones are an ester group which also has a carbon ring attached; they are some of the most anti-inflam-matory compounds known and include the essential oil arnica. Some can be stronger mucolitic agents than

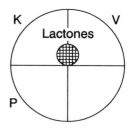

cetones; example elecampane (inula glaveolens). They are grouped with the esters on the graph.

Ethers

Ethers (sometimes called phenylpropane ethers), are very harmonizing to the nervous system. They are antiseptic, stimulant, expectorant (increase secretions), spasmolytic and diuretic. This group includes such oils as cinnamon, clove, anise, basil, tarragon, parsley, and sassafras. They are characterized by their very sweet fragrance. This group is also rather central to the chart; although somewhat more heating than the esters, their harmonizing effects have application to all doshas.

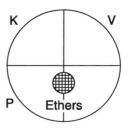

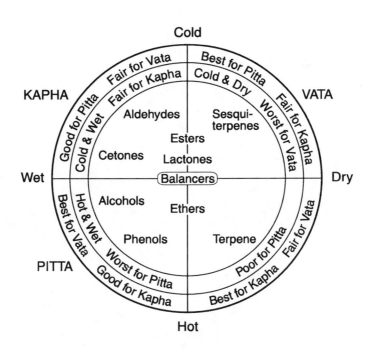

CHAPTER ELEVEN

AROMATHERAPY AND THE CORRECTION OF DOSHA IMBALANCE

*T*raditionally, Ayurveda uses plants in the form of herbs and medicated oils in treatments. For a large population, as in India, these forms have been easy to gather, make, or inexpensive to purchase. The authors assert that fresh herbs have the most complete healing properties, dried herbs and medicated oils being a close second choice. Essential oils no longer have the minerals and water-soluble components, so they are a third choice; however, they are concentrated, easy to use, and don't lose potency or spoil. In today's busy world, essential oils can be a readily available ally in healing. For balancing diet and lifestyle we recommend you consult books recommended in the bibliography. For herbal healing, the *Yoga of Herbs* is unparalleled, and we acknowledge Drs. Frawley and Lad for their approach and form in herbal healing, which we have followed in our adaptation in healing with essential oils.

ESSENTIAL OILS FOR VATA IMBALANCE

Because Vata is light, dry, mobile and cold, it is treated by the oils which are wet, heavy, calming and warming. Vata is reduced by the tastes sweet, sour and salty. There are two types of Vata imbalance to consider. One is known as obstructed Vata where the channels of the body have become clogged with toxic residues (ama), the result of indigestion, poor diet, and poor elimination in the presence of dosha imbalance. Like Kapha excess, obstructed Vata is treated for a short period of time to remove the blockages. The other type of Vata imbalance is called Vata-caused deficiency, and this is where excess Vata in the system has caused drying, emaciation and a loss of tissues. Vata-caused deficiency resembles the extreme aging process.

Obstructed Vata

For obstructed Vata, pungent essential oils are needed to remove the obstructions with heat, lightness and mobility.

Heating alteratives are used to remove accumulations of toxins and purify the blood.

ajwan	clary sage	myrrh
black pepper	coriander	saffron
calamus	cumin	sandalwood
carrot seed	dill	sassafras
cayenne	frankincense	turmeric
cinnamon	garlic	

Heating carminatives are important for normalizing and moving stuck Vata and toxins, relieving gas, normalizing digestion and for the movement of food.

ajwan	cumin	orange peel
allspice	dill	oregano
angelica	fennel	parsley
basil	galbanum	pennyroyal
bay	garlic	pine
calamus	ginger	saffron
caraway	hyssop	savory
cardamon	juniperberry	tarragon
chamomile	lavender	thyme
cinnamon	lemon	turmeric
cloves	lemon balm	valerian
coriander	lime	
cubeb	nutmeg	

Mild **warming diaphoretics** are used to induce perspiration, eliminate surface toxins, increase circulation, relieve muscle tension and aching joints, and relieve headaches due to cold or congestion.

angelica	eucalyptus	oregano
basil	fennel	pennyroyal
camphor	ginger	pine
cardamon	juniperberry	sage
chamomile	hyssop	sassafras
cinnamon	lemon balm	thyme
cloves	lemongrass	
coriander	marjoram	

Heating nervines are used to strengthen and regulate the nervous system, promote mental health, dispel intestinal gas, stop pain and clear toxins.

ajwan	fennel	nutmeg
basil	garlic	pennyroyal
calamus	lavender	sage
camphor	lemon balm	sandalwood
chamomile	marjoram	valerian
eucalyptus	myrrh	vanilla

All of these (heating carminatives, diaphoretics and nervines) may be used for a short time to remove ama; overuse can lead to drying and tissue loss, aggravating Vata.

Vata-Caused Deficiency

Vata-caused deficiency requires nutritive herbs that will build the tissues, such as **emmenagogues** and **nutritive aphrodisiacs**. These relieve menstrual cramping, build the blood, moisten and nourish the sexual immune system, strengthen organ weakness due to disease, and alleviate poor nutrition or aging.

Emmenagogues:

angelica	myrrh	rue
clary sage	parsley	saffron
galbanum	pennyroyal	tarragon
jasmine†	rose†	vanilla

† Cooling - avoid prolonged use

Aphrodisics:

aloe

Bulk and moistening laxatives would be the herbs of choice but these qualities are lost in essential oil extraction processes and are best in whole herb form. There are some essential oils such as trifolia (tumru) which, when used externally, can be **laxative**.

Moistening expectorants or **demulcents** feed the mucous membranes and strengthen, moisten and nourish the tissue. Here again, the herb form contains properties lost in essential oil production.

Nourishing tonics build the tissue, increase weight, increase vital fluids, dispel rigidity, calm the nerves and are often combined with stimulants and carminative herbs to increase absorption.

Laxative:

trifolia (tumru)

Demulcents

trifolia	jatamansi (spikenard)	tarragon
aloe	rose	

Tonics:

aloe	calamus	hops	rose
angelica	frankincense	jasmine	saffron
arnica	garlic*	jatamansi	vetiver
brahmi	Himalayan cedarwood	myrrh	

Oils for Both Types of Vata

The last group of essential oils which are good for both types of Vata are the **stimulants.** These essential oils increase digestive fire, destroy toxins, increase internal heat, and strengthen circulation. They are contraindicated for very high Vata conditions such as dehydration or inflamed mucous membranes.

ajwan	caraway	garlic*
allspice	cayenne	ginger
arnica	celery seed	marjoram
bay	cinnamon	onion*
bergamot	clove	orange
black pepper	cubeb	oregano
calamus	cumin	sassafras
camphor	eucalyptus	savory

*Please note we will mention the oils of garlic and onion; however, with the understanding that the fresh vegetable forms already contain a very high essential oil content and do not need to be concentrated in an oil form, we do not recommend the purchase or use of these essential oils. Their odors, in concentrated form, are so strong they can ruin a car or house if they are spilled. We recommend that garlic and onion be eaten in their fresh form, as foods.

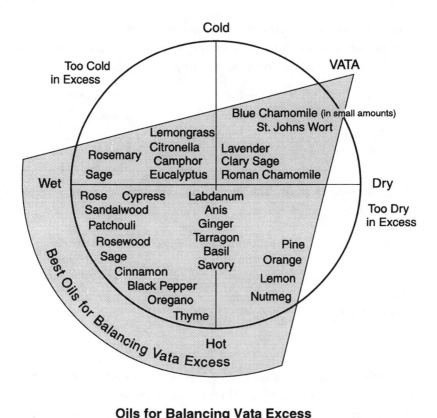

Oils for Balancing Vata Excess

ESSENTIAL OILS FOR PITTA IMBALANCE

Because Pitta is hot and wet, it is treated with cooling, heat dispelling, drying, nutritive and calming oils. The tastes for reducing Pitta are sweet, astringent, and bitter.

Cooling diaphoretic oils dispel heat from fevers or inflammatory skin conditions.

catnip	coriander	spearmint
chamomile	lemon balm	yarrow
chrysanthemum	peppermint	

99

Astringent oils reduce excretions and discharges and are drying, yet prevent the loss of moisture and have a tightening effect on tissues, promote wound healing on surface tissues, and stop bleeding.

cajeput	lemon	turmeric
calendula	saffron	wintergreen
carrot seed	St. Johns wort	yarrow

Cooling alteratives purify the blood, fight infections, reduce fevers and promote healing.

aloe vera	immortelle	sandalwood
coriander	jasmine	spearmint
cumin	keawa	tagetes
dill	neem	turmeric
henna (hina)	saffron	yarrow

Bitter tonics are strong medicine for high Pitta conditions of fever, infection, inflammation and acidity. They are used to destroy toxins or pathogens; however, overuse can lower the digestive fire and lower organ function leading to weakness and emaciation. Most are found only in herb form.

aloe vera	neem

Cooling carminatives are often aromatic spices that improve digestion and elimination by removing blockages and promoting the flow of energy.

catnip	fennel	peppermint
chamomile	lavender	saffron
chrysanthemum	lemon	spearmint
coriander	lemon balm	wintergreen
cumin	lime	
dill	neroli	

Cooling emmenagogues promote and regulate the female cycle, reduce spasms, excess bleeding, infection and anger.

carrot seed	jasmine	yarrow
chamomile	rose	
chrysanthemum	saffron	

Cooling nervines are calming to the mind and emotions and build nerve tissue.

benzoin	immortelle	peppermint
catnip	jasmine	St. Johns wort
chamomile	jatamansi	sandalwood
champa	lavender	spearmint
fennel	lemon balm	tagetes
gotu kola (brahmi)	neroli	
hina	oud	

Nutritive tonics nourish the tissues of the body, reduce inflammation, restore secretions, build the blood and the lymph system.

angelica	immortelle	neem
carrot seed	jatamansi*	neroli
cedarwood	musk	spikenard

*Heating: avoid excessive use or use during Pitta excess

Rejuvenatives renew the body and mind, increase awareness, change patterns, create expansion.

angelica	hina	rose
brahmi	jatamansi	saffron
carrot seed	musk	
cedarwood	oud	

Cooling diuretics reduce Pitta's heat, and cool the liver.

benzoin	lavender	spearmint
coriander	lemongrass	
fennel	sandalwood	

Antipyretics reduce Pitta's fire.

benzoin	jasmine	neroli
champa	keawa	tagetes
hina	lime	vetiver
immortelle	neem	

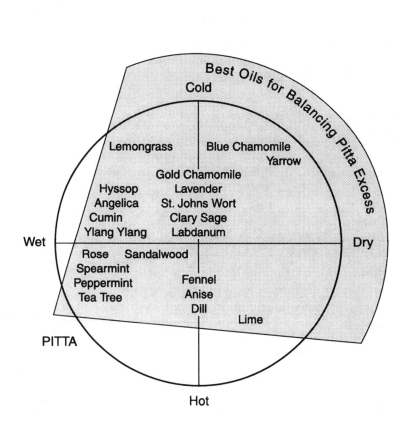

Oils for Balancing Pitta Excess

ESSENTIAL OILS FOR KAPHA IMBALANCE

Because Kapha is water and earth, it is predominately cold, moist, slow and heavy in nature. It can be treated with warming, drying, lightening and stimulating therapy. The tastes that improve or balance Kapha are pungent, bitter and astringent. Pungent is the most important because it is exactly opposite from Kapha, being light, hot and dry.

Diuretics can be used to reduce water and are an important Kapha therapy.

ajwan	fennel	parsley
cinnamon	garlic	spearmint
coriander	juniperberry	
cubeb	lemongrass	

The main areas that hold Kapha energy (in the form of mucous) are the lungs and the stomach. Emetic therapy is important for expelling mucous buildups in the stomach and the lungs but should only be administered by those who have special knowledge and training (see pancha karma, page 199).

Diaphoretic oils can be helpful for eliminating water through sweating. They cleanse the blood and lymphatics.

ajwan	cloves	onion
angelica	eucalyptus	oregano
basil	ginger	sage
camphor	juniperberry	sassafras
cardamon	lemongrass	thyme
cinnamon	mugwort	

Cooling diaphoretics, because they promote cleansing, are good for Kapha (unless experiencing a cold or flu).

catnip †	coriander†	yarrow†
chamomile†	peppermint†	
chrysanthemum†	spearmint†	

Increasing the digestive fire reduces Kapha, so all stimulant and **carminative** essential oils can be important therapy, especially the heating carminatives and stimulants.

ajwan	cloves	oregano
anise	cubeb	parsley
basil	elecampane	pennyroyal
bay	garlic	saffron
black pepper	ginger	thyme
calamus	juniperberry	turmeric
cardamon	mustard	valerian
cayenne	nutmeg	
cinnamon	orange peel	

Even **cooling carminatives** can help stimulate Kapha's digestion.

chamomile†	cumin†	peppermint†
catnip†	dill†	sandalwood
chrysanthemum†	fennel†	spearmint†
coriander†	lime†	wintergreen†

†Cooling: avoid excessive or prolonged use.

Stimulant and **digestive** oils increase the metabolism.

ajwan	cloves	ginger
anise	coriander	juniperberry
bay	cubeb	mustard
black pepper	cumin	orange peel
camphor	damiana	oregano
cardamon	eucalyptus	pennyroyal
cayenne	fennel	sassafras
cinnamon	garlic	turmeric

Bitter tonics will reduce Kapha and are important for reducing the cravings for sweets. Most are found only in herb form.

neem

Aromatic **heating nervines** will stimulate the nervous activity, clear channels and relieve congestion.

basil	eucalyptus	nutmeg
bayberry	garlic	pennyroyal
calamus	mugwort	sage
camphor	myrrh	valerian

Cooling nervines

chamomile†	peppermint†	St. Johns wort†
gotu kola (brahmi)†	rose†	yarrow†
jasmine†	sandalwood†	
jatamansi†	spearmint†	

†Cooling: avoid excessive or prolonged use.

Laxative essential oils help to reduce the earth element.

trifolia, external application   parsley

Nutritive tonics increase Kapha because they are composed primarily of earth and water and are generally uncalled for with the exception of:

angelica	gotu kola (brahmi)	onion
dhavana	jatamansi	saffron
elecampane	myrrh	

Aphrodisiacs will stimulate the sexual endocrine system.

angelica	garlic	onion
clove	jasmine	rose
damiana	nutmeg	saffron

Alteratives are good for Kapha because they cleanse the blood and lymph of impurities.

black pepper	dill	rose
cayenne	garlic	saffron
chrysanthemum	hibiscus	sandalwood
cinnamon	jasmine	sassafras
coriander	myrrh	turmeric
cumin	neem	

Astringent oils reduces Kapha's water and congestion.

black pepper	hibiscus	rose	St. Johns wort
cayenne	jasmine	saffron	turmeric
cinnamon	juniperberry	sage	wintergreen
ginger	nutmeg	sandalwood	yarrow

Heating emmenagogues build the female immune system.

angelica	mugwort	saffron
cinnamon	mustard	sage
ginger	myrrh	turmeric
hibiscus	parsley	valerian
jasmine	pennyroyal	

Cooling emmenagogues

chamomile†	rose†	yarrow†

†Cooling: avoid excessive or prolonged use.

Tonic and **rejuvenatives**

angelica	hibiscus	rose
brahmi	jasmine	saffron

Expectorant and demulcent oils clear out the bronchioles, sinus and cleanse the mucous membranes.

ajwan	clove	hyssop
bay	cubeb	jatamansi
black pepper	dill	lime
calamus	elecampane	mustard
camphor	garlic	orange peel
cardamon	ginger	sage
cinnamon	hibiscus	St. Johns wort

For cough relief

eucalyptus   thyme

So almost all essential oils are good for Kapha. Of course, the warming and drying oils will be best.

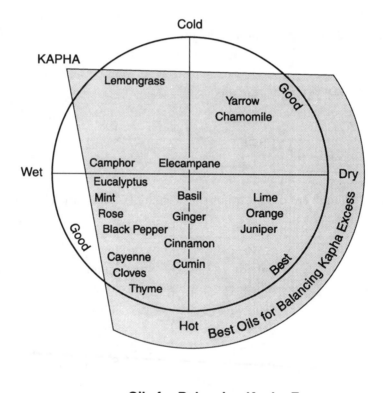

Oils for Balancing Kapha Excess

SECTION III

APPLICATIONS OF ESSENTIAL OILS

CHAPTER TWELVE

AYURVEDIC BLENDING

Blending is the art of putting two or
more essential oils together for a synergistic effect. An important principal of
blending is to avoid using opposites, as one oil will negate the effects of the
other. For example, if you were to blend oils for calming or cooling the
environment, it would be contradictory to add a heating, stimulating essential oil to your mixture.

The French method of blending divides the oils into two axes of opposing qualities. On the left/right axis they have narcotic and stimulating oils.
On the up/down axis they have fresh and clean at the top, and erogenous at
the bottom. Each of these are opposing factors; oils which have strong stimulating qualities should not be mixed with oils which have narcotic qualities.
Narcotic is the opposite of stimulating, clean is the opposite of erogenous;
oils of opposing characteristics will cancel each other out if mixed together.
By understanding this, the blender can avoid this unfortunate occurrence.
Dr. Kurt Schnaubelt, in his aromatherapy course, beautifully presents this
method of blending, and shows that clean or anti-erogenous oil, mixed with
stimulating, becomes refreshing; stimulating oil mixed with erogenous becomes exalting; erogenous oil mixed with narcotic becomes sultry; and narcotic oil mixed with anti-erogenous becomes calming. When I first saw this
chart, I suddenly understood what perfume descriptions were talking about
when they spoke of exalting and sultry, etc. For those who want to know

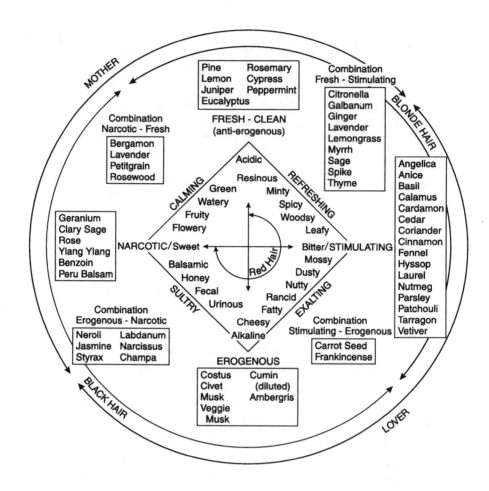

Adapted from Aromatherapy Correspondence Course, Kurt Schnaubelt.

The French Perfume Blending Method

more about this method of blending, I would refer you to Dr. Schnaubelt's study course (see Resource Guide).

There are many other methods of blending, including astrological blending for certain signs of the Zodiac, for the planets, the elements, even the Kabala. For this blending I would refer you to *The Magical and Ritual Use of Perfumes* by Richard Allen Miller and Iona Miller (no relation to the authors). They also describe a blending method by an Italian researcher named Paresse who arranged a number of the essential oils along a musical scale based on evaporation rates (the speed with which essential oils evaporate). Chords can be formed with these arrangements of notes which theoretically should be harmonious. For instance, the bouquet of Chord C would include, going from bass to treble: sandalwood, geranium, acacia, orange flower and camphor.

Notes

One of the most common ways of blending essential oils in aromatherapy is based upon evaporation rates. All oils are divided into top, middle and base notes, according to their rate of evaporation.

Top Notes are oils with fast evaporation rates that come to your nose very quickly. They are what you first smell about an essential oil and often are the strongest, but unfortunately leave most quickly. Citrus oils are famous for their top notes. Top notes compose 10-15% of the total blend. Their fast evaporation is explained by very high terpene content (terpenes being small molecules which evaporate quickly). A drop placed on blotter paper allows the oil to diffuse with the top note disappearing typically in 15 minutes to 2 hours.

Middle notes are often the second aroma you encounter after the rush of the top note has disappeared. They form the body of the blend. Typically, they are 40-80% of the oil blend and are responsible for blending the sharp smell of the top note with the deepness of the base notes. The middle notes are usually derived from the group of plants we would call herbs; rosewood, lavender, chamomile, geranium. They are typically warm, soft, mellow, balancers and equalizers. Often these work with the middle portion of the body's metabolism, including its digestion and organ functions, whereas the top notes work most strongly with the mind. The middle notes can be detected on blotter paper from several hours to several days.

The **base notes** are known as the fixatives, because they fix or hold the smell and slow down or draw out the evaporative rate of the top notes. Typical base notes would be patchouli, cedarwood, and vetiver. Often these oils are thick and dark. Smelling them from the bottle, they often don't smell that strong, but once the heat of the body or diffuser releases them, their smell is tenacious, often lasting several days. Base notes often have an unpleasant odor but are extremely important, even if they comprise no more than 5% of the blend. Base notes have a long history of spiritual usage (anointing the chakras) and often have an affinity with the male or female sexual organs. Base notes can remain evident on paper from several days to weeks.

It is important to remember that essential oils contain hundreds of chemical components. Some of these components will be top notes, others middle notes or base notes. For example, angelica is known for a very strong top note which comes quickly to the nose (it is a musk cetone of small molecular size), but angelica also has middle and base notes associated with it. Many times an oil is a complete blend in itself, carrying the full range of smells. Rose is another good example, having both high, middle and base notes.

When reading essential oil and aromatherapy books, you may become confused because one person lists a particular oil as a top note, another person lists it as a middle note, and sometimes both are correct.

The value in blending an oil mixture is that you may achieve several effects at once. In dealing with acne, for instance, you may want your oil blend to have disinfectant qualities because of the opportunistic bacteria which are causing irritation on the skin surface. This requirement could be satisfied with an oil such as lavender. You may also want an essential oil that can decrease the skin's oil production and be calming to the skin's metabolism. You might choose an oil like carrot seed or cedarwood for this purpose. Inflammation can sometimes be a component of acne, so an anti-inflammatory oil such as St. Johns wort or blue chamomile may be appropriate. Many people feel that acne can be a reflection of inner disturbance, low self-esteem, or lack of assurance, so you may choose an oil like angelica for its psychological property of giving inner strength. So the blender's job is to look at all these different possibilities, select oils that will work together synergistically and not oppose each other energetically; make sure the oil blend is well rounded, having top, middle and base notes; and is pleasant-smelling. Often the purpose of a top or middle note is to cover up an unpleasant, but therapeutically important, base oil.

To all of this traditional art of blending you can add consideration for Ayurvedic types and conditions caused by dosha imbalance. We (the authors) have taken our Vata, Pitta and Kapha oils and divided each category into top, middle and base notes to assist the Ayurvedic aromatherapist in creating well balanced Ayurvedic blends. It is recommended that you:

1. pick the dosha imbalance for which you are blending,

2. pick the oils which have therapeutic qualities in top, middle and base note categories for the dosha imbalance,

3. experiment in small quantities (drops), using the following percentage guidelines: 10-15% top notes, 40-80% middle notes, and 5% base notes, and

4. when you have a blend that smells nice and meets your therapeutic needs, you may make it in larger quantities.

5. example: 2 drops angelica, 10 drops chamomile, and 1 drop myrrh, in 1/4 oz. vegetable oil.

Blending Oils for Vata

TOP	MIDDLE	BASE
allspice	ajwan	angelica (top & base)
angelica	bay	calamus
anise	cardamon	carrot seed
arnica	chamomile	cinnamon
basil	cinnamon	(base to middle)
bergamot	clary sage	cloves
camphor	(top & middle)	cumin
clary sage	coriander	frankincense
cubeb	dill	galbanum
eucalyptus	fennel	ginger
lemon	hops	jatamansi
myrtle	lavender	myrrh
orange	nutmeg	rose
pine	rosewood	trifolia
tangerine	tarragon	
	vanilla	

Blending Oils for Pitta

TOP	MIDDLE	BASE
bergamot	brahmi	calendula
champa	clary sage	cumin
lemon	coriander	hina
lemongrass	dill	jasmine
lime	fennel	myrrh
orange	hina	neem
wintergreen	hops	rose
	mace	sandalwood
	peppermint	tarragon
	saffron	turmeric
	St. Johns wort	valerian
	spearmint	vanilla
	turmeric	vetiver

Blending Oils for Kapha

TOP	MIDDLE	BASE
basil	ajwan	angelica
camphor	anise	calamus
champa	bay	cardamon
cubeb	black pepper	cinnamon
elecampane	chamomile	clove
elemi	cinnamon	cumin
lemon	clary sage	cypress
lemongrass	coriander	dhavana
lime	dill	garlic
niaouli	ginger	Himalayan cedarwood
orange	hyssop	jasmine
pine	juniper	jatamansi
	oregano	myrrh
	parsley	neem
	peppermint	neroli
	rosemary	nutmeg
	thyme	rose
		sage
		sandalwood
		trifolia
		turmeric
		valerian

Carrier Oils

The vegetable oil that you use in making your ayurvedic blends can be as important as the essential oils which you choose. Each vegetable oil has individual characteristics which can be important in determining choices.

Carrier Oils for Vata Reduction Blends:

(– : lowers dosha)
(+ : increases dosha)
(o : neutral)
(= : good for all doshas, balancing)

Because vata is dry, all oils are potentially good.

Avocado oil (VK– P+) is sweet and warm, excellent for the liver, high in vitamin E, is a skin moisturizer, and is good for weak tissues.

Castor oil (VK– P+) is thick, warm and sweet, excellent for constipation and dry stools when used internally; it helps to relieve muscle spasm and arthritic pain in compress form, and helps stimulate movement of the lymph.

Flax oil (VK– P+) helps with constipation and dryness, is high in essential fatty acids and so is stimulating to the system. Excellent for internal use.

Peanut oil (V– KP+) is warm, sweet and strong smelling. It is difficult to cover up its own aroma with essential oils, but was heavily used by Edgar Cayce for its curative properties.

Sesame oil (V– PK+) is excellent for dry skin. It is nourishing and protective (it blocks up to 45% of the sun's UV rays) and is high in minerals.

Walnut oil (V– KP+) is cooling, calming to the skin, excellent for infections; it has a rather strong smell so is not preferred for delicate blends, but can be highly nutritious and nourishing because of its source.

Carrier Oils for Pitta Reduction Blends:

Coconut oil (P– K+ Vo) is cooling, excellent for sun tan lotion (it helps reflect radiation), is a skin moisturizer, helps inflammation, skin infections, and contrary to common belief, it does not have any aroma unless synthetic fragrance has been added.

Olive oil (P– K+) is sweet and neutral, and is probably one of the best oils for softening gall stones and decongesting the bile system; it has antiseptic and stimulant properties, is excellent for joint pain, and to make medicated oils. Its somewhat strong smell makes it less popular for massage blends.

Sunflower oil (PK– Vo) is sweet and cool, nourishing, good for rashes and infections.

Carrier Oils for Kapha Reduction Blends:

Canola oil (KV– P+) is low in saturated fats and helps the skin to maintain youthfulness. In the mustard family, it helps to bring heat to the formulas.

Corn oil (KV– P+) is highly diuretic, brings warmth, and is excellent for edema and swelling.

Mustard oil (KV– P+) is often found in Oriental and Indian grocery stores. It is pungent and hot, helping to break down congested tissue; can be especially good for compresses on the lungs and is good for abdominal pain.

Safflower oil (VK– P+) is warm and pungent, excellent for pregnancy, normal skin, circulatory problems, female complaints.

Soy oil (PK– Vo) is astringent, has drying properties, and contains vitamins A and E which help preserve and maintain a healthy glow to the skin.

Sweet almond oil (VK– P+) is also heating and a favorite of massage therapists because of its mild smell. Avoid bitter almond—it is used in small amounts as a flavoring, but applied to the skin it can be poisonous and irritating.

Oils for All Types

Aloe Vera oil (VPK=) is actually a medicated oil which you can make yourself by slicing up the leaves of the fresh aloe vera plant, placing them in a glass jar and covering with vegetable oil. Allow the mixture to soak for 30 to 60 days then strain. Any vegetable oil can be enhanced by adding aloe vera (or any healing herb) to make your own medicated oils.

Apricot kernel oil (VKP=) is a favorite with massage therapists. It is sweet, warming, clean, not strong smelling. Makes the skin feel lustrous and adds a healthy glow. It is used in India for medicinal purposes to help constipation and infections.

Hazelnut oil (VKP=) is warming and nourishing, good for dry irritated skin, has a strong nutty fragrance.

Jojoba oil (VPK=) is expressed from the fruit of a plant that grows in the American Southwest. I recall hiking in Arizona and eating the small fruits as I went along the trail. Jojoba oil is actually a wax and so it does not spoil or become rancid as other vegetable oils do. It has anti-inflammatory properties, it is good for the hair, and it is often used in skin care formulas as it has sun-screen properties and contains many vitamins and minerals. "Unrefined" jojoba oil has a somewhat strong, almost nutty, smell; in our blends we prefer "refined," which is clear and has almost no fragrance.

Primrose oil (PVK=) is a wonderful oil to use for phytoestrogen (plant estrogen) patches, it is extremely immune-system building because of its essential fatty acid content, and is very expensive, as much as $100 for 8 ounces (wholesale). It is almost a waste to use it externally.

Wheatgerm oil (VPK=) is too expensive to use as a blend in itself but can be added to all blends (1 part in 10) to add shelf life because of its anti-oxidant qualities.

CHAPTER THIRTEEN

PERSONAL CARE

THE BATH

Light: One of my favorite ways to use essential oils is in the bath. Rarely do I start the day without taking an essential oil bath. While the water is running, I brush my skin with a dry skin brush in a circular motion towards the heart. This is also a good time to say affirmations.

When the bath is ready, I put 15-30 drops of my favorite oils in the tub and step in. I usually select oils that are good for my body type. Depending on what I ate the night before, my Kapha nature may be activated in the mornings, causing water retention. If so, I use 5 drops cypress, 5 drops juniperberry, and 5 drops orange in the bath.

When my Vata is activated (by doing too much or staying up too late), I may wake up spacey and disconnected. I then use 5 drops rosewood, 5 drops jatamansi, and 5 drops yarrow.

In very hot weather, or if my Pitta is up, I may use 5 drops lavender, 5 drops sandalwood, and 5 drops champa. Of course you can choose your favorite oils to balance your doshic type.

Bathing is a way to take time for yourself, take time to relax and connect with life forces. It is wonderful to combine the bath with meditation—nothing is more relaxing and rejuvenating. What a wonderful way to start your day.

INHALATION

When under stress, people often feel stuck in depression, anger, fear, and anxiety, and may experience loss of memory and lack of creativity. Inhalation (breathing in) of essential oils can most deeply affect these emotional states.

Poor diet and over-consumption of dairy products may cause sinus problems, headaches, congestion, and many other symptoms that can be relieved by inhalation. Inhalation brings essential oils in vapor form to the mucous membranes of the upper respiratory tract, calming, opening, and fighting invaders.

Inhalation is one of the fastest ways to bring change and transformation to thoughts and feelings, as inhalation of essential oils stimulates the limbic system (that most primitive part of our brain, storing memories, emotions, and desires), and brings about the immediate release of hormones and neurotransmitters. What better way to transform ourselves than to "breathe in" (inhale) appropriate essential oils. Inspiration, after all, means "breathing in of spirit."

How to Practice Inhalation

The best way to practice inhalation is to purchase an inhalation device. The old method is to boil water, pour it into a bowl, and put in 3 to 5 drops of essential oil; if you are using heating oils such as thyme or eucalyptus, you may want to use only 2 drops. Make sure the water is steaming, put a towel over your head, close your eyes, and take slow, deep breaths. Be careful not to get too close to the steam. You will notice a diminishing odor after three minutes. At that time you can add more essential oils or terminate the treatment. For acute illness, allergic

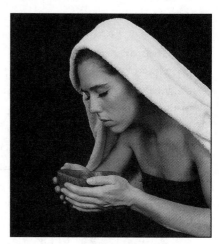

Inhalation

reaction, or hay fever, do an inhalation treatment every fifteen minutes. For more chronic conditions (mucous congestion, depression), perform an inhalation every two to four hours. Reduce frequency as symptoms diminish.

A Good Combination of Oils for:

Colds	Flu	Depression	Sinusitis	Cough	Fever
two drops each	one drop each	two drops each	one drop each	one drop each	two drops lavender
eucalyptus rosemary camphor	thyme cajeput	bergamot geranium lemongrass	angelica eucalyptus neroli cypress yarrow	hyssop sage anise sandalwood	one drop chamomile

As 95% of our illnesses start in our emotional bodies, almost any condition can be treated with inhalation of essential oils.

COMPRESS

Light: I have memories of lying in bed as a child with a hot compress relaxing my breathing. I had an asthma condition from the stress of changing homes and much traveling. Warm compresses help open the pores and allow the volatile oils to penetrate the skin and go into the tissue. Essential oils penetrate the skin two hundred times faster than water. For a compress, mix 5 to 10 drops of essential oils in about a quart of hot water. Then immerse a small towel or piece of flannel in the water, squeeze most of the water out after soaking a few minutes, and apply on the area of complaint. Add a heating pad or hot water bottle to assist in the penetration of the oil and to keep the compress warm.

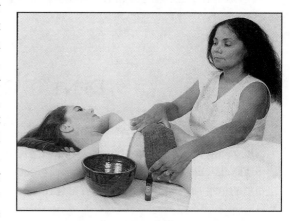

Compress

Cold Compress

While living in Hawaii, we were visited by a young woman from the Pacific Northwest. She had beautiful, white porcelain-like skin, and was horrified to find that, with only a few days of over exposure to the strong tropical sun, she was suffering broken red capillaries on the side of her nose. She was given a recipe for a cold compress, utilizing one drop of rose oil (only the best distilled) and one drop of parsley seed oil mixed into one-half cup of cool water. She applied this mixture to the broken capillaries for fifteen minutes twice a day. A cold pack or crushed ice in a plastic bag was placed over the compress to keep it cool. She wrote several months later to report that it took about two weeks for the capillaries to disappear, and that she was ecstatic to have her beautiful skin back.

When using compresses for specific conditions, remember that pain is usually an indication of Vata imbalance. Because **Vata** is cold, you will want to use a warm compress. **Pitta** conditions are usually characterized by redness, inflammation and heat. On areas of Pitta imbalance, cool or cold compresses are best. **Kapha** conditions are characterized by lack of fluid movement, swelling and congestion. Here again, warm or hot compresses are best.

When placing a compress on an organ, if the organ is overactive, a cool compress is best; if underactive, use a warm compress. For example, with liver or gall bladder congestion, you may use 5 drops of rosemary and 5 drops of coriander, and heat. A Pitta person may use a cool compress of coriander. For Kapha, use ginger and rosemary, and heat.

DENTAL CARE

We think that our teeth decay only from poor diet or hygiene. Recently, I discovered they decay faster while we are under stress. Brushing with essential oils can be very beneficial to preserve and maintain healthy gums. Use one drop on your toothbrush each time you brush.

Vata	Pitta	Kapha
neem oil	peppermint	fennel
myrrh	angelica	sage
cypress	geranium	rosemary
	lavender	bergamot

SKIN CARE

Essential oils penetrate deeply into the layers of the skin, affecting not only the surface of the skin, but they also absorb into the capillaries, becoming a part of the whole person, physiologically and psychologically. Ayurveda sees essential oils as pure prana from the plant; the plant's gift to us for the purpose of nourishing, cleansing, detoxifying, increasing circulation, toning, calming nerve irritation and supporting all the skin's function.

There are only a few essential oils that can be used directly on the skin, and this can be done because the skin has a natural oil mantle (covering). When you rub one drop of essential oil into the skin you are really rubbing it into the natural oil that is already there, so you are diluting it. Chamomile, lavender, rose, sandalwood and yarrow are all oils that can be used, one drop directly on the skin. People with sensitive skin need to be careful, though people with tougher skin may even use strong oils such as rosemary in very small amounts, without adverse effect. The general rule is that essential oils should always be diluted before applying to the skin.

Essential oils may be added to your current skin cream or lotion, or you can purchase your skin creams unscented and add specific essential oils for your particular needs. You can choose a vegetable oil that is appropriate for your skin and add specific essential oils to create a moisturizing oil that's just for you. **Vata** does best with all vegetable oils, but especially with sesame and hazelnut. **Pitta** is more sensitive; olive, sunflower and coconut being the most cooling. **Kapha** needs the least oil of all, but can do best with heating oils such as almond or mustard seed. All skin types do very well with jojoba. Because jojoba is actually a wax, it is particularly useful because it does not become rancid. Any skin product which you make with jojoba oil will have a longer shelf-life and you will not need to refrigerate it between uses.

Vegetable oil mixtures that you will use within a month do not need to be refrigerated, but any product you use infrequently and hope to keep for six months should be refrigerated between use, just as you refrigerate vegetable oils that you cook with.

Never apply any product with a rancid smell to your skin. There may be an inner voice which says, "Do not waste this, I paid for this, use it," but rancid oils contain, or cause the release of, free radicals, which cause aging, create stress for the immune system, and should be avoided at all costs, even if it means throwing out an expensive mixture.

It is possible to preserve your oil mixtures by using 3 to 5 drops of benzoin per one-half ounce. You can also squeeze a vitamin E capsule into the solution, add wheat germ oil or vitamin E oil, 3 to 5 drops per ounce. Essential oils have preservative qualities in themselves; the stronger your mixture, is the less tendency it will have to go rancid. It is still recommended to refrigerate oils that have been enhanced with these above-mentioned products, just for safety.

The Structure of the Skin

The skin is a very elaborate defense mechanism created to protect the body from invasion and loss of moisture. It grows from inside out, progressively pushing older layers of skin cells toward the surface. As these skin cells get farther and farther away from their source of capillary nourishment, they die; so the top three layers of skin are composed of dead cells, and this thick layer of compact dead cells acts as a barrier to invasion of bacteria or virus. The outer layer of dead cells is constantly being shed and replaced by the next layer pushing up. Skin brushing, or using a luffa sponge, can greatly enhance the removal of these old cells and provide a stimulation to the formation of new cells underneath.

The acid mantle of the skin is composed of oil and sebum, excreted by the sebaceous glands, and helps to form a protective layer which holds moisture and protects against invasion. Soaps are generally of an alkaline nature and will strip away the acid mantle of the skin. This is why healthcare experts recommend against the use of soaps or shampoos which have not been PH balanced. PH balance varies from individual to individual but should be somewhere around 4.5 to 5.5 PH (on the acid side of neutral).

Because essential oils penetrate through the outer layers of skin to the nerve endings, capillaries, sebaceous glands, and hair follicles, they can beneficially affect all the skin functions. Essential oils can increase or decrease oil excretion onto the skin, stimulate the circulatory system to produce more surface warmth, or slow the circulatory system to cool inflammation.

Because of essential oils' antiviral, antibacterial, antifungal characteristics, when they become a part of the acid mantle of the skin, they assist in protecting against these invading organisms.

Some skin conditions can be created by nervous over-stimulation or lack of nerve impulses. Many essential oils can assist in providing balance to the nervous system.

Our hormones affect our skin; an excess of male hormone contributes to deep cysts and other forms of acne. Many of the essential oils which increase estrogen production can help to correct conditions of this type.

It is important to remember that it takes forty days for new skin cells to be pushed out to the surface of the skin. Any program you undertake to correct a skin condition will need that much time in order to be properly evaluated.

The skin is also an excretory organ, eliminating up to one-quarter of all our body metabolic wastes. It is a good practice to make sure the old dead cells are removed through essential oil baths and skin brushing to assist in waste removal. If the skin is blocked and wastes are not removed via this outlet, the toxic load will have to be carried by the other eliminative organs such as the liver, the kidneys and the lungs.

Many essential oils stimulate perspiration (diaphoretics), most notable of which are yarrow, ginger, juniper, rosemary, and eucalyptus.

Vata skin is characterized by dryness, flaking, cracking, wrinkling, thinness, coldness, roughness, and can be assisted by such Vata-reducing essential oils as chamomile, clary sage, geranium, lavender, jasmine, jatamansi, rose, rosewood, sandalwood and vetiver.

Pitta skin is characterized by irritations, acne, and sensitivity and can be assisted by such essential oils as blue chamomile, geranium, jasmine, lavender, rose, rosewood, sandalwood, peppermint. When Pitta skin becomes oily it can be assisted by such essential oils as bergamot, camphor, cedarwood, cypress, geranium, juniperberry, lavender, lemon, rosewood, sandalwood and vetiver, all of which decrease oil secretion.

Kapha skin is often smooth, normal and thick, but occasionally can experience lack of blood flow, so a slight coolness and buildup of edema can be assisted with birch, clary sage, cypress, orange, rosemary, eucalyptus and juniperberry.

Mature and aging skin can affect any dosha type and can be assisted with the use of blue chamomile, clary sage, cypress, frankincense, lavender, fennel, neroli, orange, rose, rosewood, sandalwood, vetiver.

Cellulite is a special problem which is thought to be a buildup of toxins in the skin that causes a peculiar orange-peel-type puckering. By the theory of signatures used in herbs, any plant that resembles the condition in the human is helpful for that condition; therefore, orange peel essential oil is useful in cellulite as would be birch, cypress, juniperberry, lemon and rosemary.

Cysts are thought to be caused by an excess of male hormone, which produces a cellular irritation and an increased cell division, creating smaller, more numerous cells. As they are pushed upward to the skin surface, the result is flaking and cracking. This condition can be assisted with bergamot, clary sage, lavender, frankincense, geranium and especially neem.

Whereas **dry skin** is a Vata condition, it can occur in any dosha type, especially in dry climates such as the American southwest. All dosha types in this climate may need to take on the Vata regimen of oiling the skin as much as three times a day. While this may seem a bother, the alternative is to have dry, cracked, prematurely aged, wrinkled skin. We grew up worshipping the sun and I remember some of my mother's friends who sunbathed until they had a beautiful dark tan every year. As they got older, their skin wrinkled and sagged much more than my mother, who enjoyed sitting in the shade, reading.

For **broken capillaries**: German chamomile, rose, neroli, lavender, parsley seed oil, and rosewood.

In addition to lotions, creams and body oils, beeswax salve, applied to special problem areas, can be especially good for preventing moisture loss.

Essential Oil Salves

Salve is the combining of the healing power of herbs with the preservation and penetration properties of vegetable oil, hardened by the addition of beeswax. The more wax added to a mixture, the firmer it becomes. The more oil, the softer it becomes. Consideration should be made as to the outside temperatures where the salve will be used. A salve for backpacking in the Arizona desert in summer may need to have more beeswax in it than a salve made for skiing in Colorado in the winter.

The basic recipe for salve is one part beeswax to four to six parts of medicated vegetable oil. Medicated vegetable oil is made much like medicated ghee, by soaking herbs in vegetable oil for thirty to sixty days, then straining to remove the herbs. Of course, the addition of essential oils will quickly make your vegetable oil medicated.

Using a small pan or pot (stainless steel preferable, ceramic acceptable, Teflon discouraged), slowly melt the beeswax, add the estimated amount of vegetable oil, and stir until well blended. To check the consistency, take a cold spoon out of the freezer (which you placed there earlier) and dip into your mixture. The salve will instantly harden on the spoon. At this point, if it is too hard, add more oil. If it is too soft, add more beeswax. Take the pan off the heat as soon as everything is melted, and put it back on the heat only if it begins to harden too much. Once you have the consistency you desire, you can combine various essential oils and add 20 to 40 drops to one ounce of salve. Wheat germ oil and benzoin can be added as a preservative, or you can squeeze a capsule of vitamin E into the mixture. Stir and pour into a wide-mouth container, baby food jar, recycled cosmetics container, etc.

Burn Salve - 5 drops lavender, 5 drops blue chamomile, 5 drops gold chamomile, 5 drops yarrow.

Antiseptic Salve - 3 drops pine, 5 drops lavender, 7 drops eucalyptus, 7 drops rosemary.

Antifungal Salve - 10 drops thyme, 10 drops yarrow, 10 drops chamomile (This particular mixture is interesting because it might seem contradictory to use thyme and chamomile, since one is heating and one is cooling. Both are very antifungal, however, and since the intent of the therapy is not to produce heat or cold, but to fight fungus and yeast, their combination is acceptable in this case.

Mental Clarity Salve to be rubbed on the forehead - 10 drops rosemary, 10 drops basil, 5 drops chamomile, 5 drops mint.

Have fun making up your own combinations.

HAIR CARE

The hair and scalp are actually just part of the skin. Many of the things which applied to skin care apply to hair care, including having acid-balanced hair care products.

For **hair loss**, essential oils of birch, brahmi, chamomile, coriander, peppermint, rose and rosewood. This is symptomatic of Pitta excess.

For **oily hair** (also Pitta) it is recommended to use cedar, lavender, lemon, sage, lemon balm and cypress.

For **graying hair** (Pitta-Vata), coriander, sage and lemon can halt the progress.

To **increase hair growth**, rosemary, coriander, cedar and birch.

For Vata **split ends**, rosewood, sandalwood and vetiver.

For Vata **dandruff** lavender, yarrow, sandalwood, lemon balm, bay, lemon, neem, and cypress.

Bryan: One of my favorite ways to add essential oils to my scalp and hair is to buy a good, natural, PH-balanced shampoo and separate conditioner. In a four-ounce bottle of each, I will add approximately twenty to thirty drops of a synergistic blend of essential oils.

Ayurvedic treatment for the scalp includes nightly oiling with appropriately medicated vegetable oils.

RECIPES

Hair loss	**Dandruff**
To 4 oz. coconut oil, add:	To 4 oz. sesame oil, add:
10 drops chamomile	10 drops lavender
10 drops coriander	10 drops yarrow
10 drops rosewood	10 drops cypress
10 drops birch	10 drops sandalwood

ENVIRONMENTAL FRAGRANCING

Today we are very fortunate to have so many ways to disperse essential oils into the air. Aromatherapy rings rest on top of light bulbs, using that source of heat. There are electric diffusers which use aquarium pumps to force air and essential oils into a fine mist; however, in many of the aromatherapy diffusers, the aquarium pump makes a background noise which may be annoying. There is a new type of diffuser which utilizes a cotton wick saturated with water and essential oils, and a silent fan which diffuses the oils into the room. With an aromatherapy lamp (potpourri pot), you can create magic just by lighting a candle. You can bring the aromas of nature into your home all day.

When the children were small and they came home with colds, we would immediately light an aromatherapy lamp in their play room, using rosemary and eucalyptus oils.

A vaporizer is a great way to diffuse oils and to put moisture and a wonderful aroma into a dry room. Just add 10-15 drops of oils into the water. If you burn a wood stove, place a pot of water on top and periodically add essential oils. In the winter, it is especially important to add moisture and oils to the dry, overheated air.

One of the fastest and easiest ways to environmentally fragrance a room is to use a spritzer or spray bottle. These are easy to obtain but unfortunately most of them do not contain components in their pump mechanism which can withstand essential oils, even in dilution. We have bought dozens of pretty plastic spray bottles in grocery and drug stores, only to have them fail, sometimes in a matter of days. For a bit more money, you can buy a spray bottle which is resistant to chemicals. Try a garden shop. The intended use for these sprayers is for pesticides and herbicides, and they're not beautiful (with all kinds of information, warnings and technical information on them). However, you can spray-paint the bottles with your favorite color, or glue some pretty cloth or

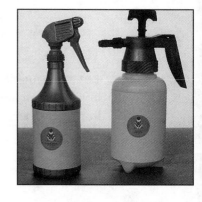

Fragrancing Bottles

paper around the outside. These will work with your ordinary dilutions of essential oils. In a quart of water, 15-30 drops is generally more than sufficient, and you'll be surprised how long that quart will last, and at the dramatic change in the environment. Plants love to be spritzed, and the essential oils in your spray bottle only add more life to them as long as your mixtures are well-diluted. Plants will be happy to take in the essential oil from one of their brothers and use it in their own defense and immune systems.

Some people use these sprays to encourage fleas to leave their pets, using mixtures that insects don't like—such as pennyroyal, sage, eucalyptus, tea tree, and citronella. I would recommend doing this outside, so that if the fleas jump off, they will not be jumping off in your house. Be sure to protect your pet's eyes from the spray.

You can drop a few drops of essential oils into the wax of a burning candle, and as the candle draws the oil up into it's wick, the essential oils will be released (the burning alters their smell somewhat). You can also do this with oil lamps.

It is possible to add essential oils to incense. Nag Champa, which is one of my favorite types of incense, is made from the bark of the champa tree. But you can add champa flower oil onto the incense before you light it. Other favorite incense additives would be sandalwood, camphor, jatamansi, rose and cinnamon.

The number of ways to add essential oils into the environment is only limited by our imagination. Sophisticated diffusion systems for industrial use have been developed, in which quantities of essential oils are diffused into air conditioning systems and circulated throughout whole buildings. These are being marketed and used around the world, especially in Japan. Increased work efficiency has been documented when workers are exposed to changing essential oil aromas every 15 to 20 minutes.

SENSUAL ENHANCEMENT — APHRODISIA

"One man's aphrodisiac is another man's disappointment."

Tantra teaches that each one of us has a sensuous, ecstatic nature covered up by guilt, shame, and unexpressed emotions. To tap this primal nature, there is no panacea; however, you can use your understanding of the nature of metabolic types to select essential oils for use in diffusions, baths, perfume oils, body oils, sachets (or drops on pillow), and inclusion in food and drink.

Essential oils which are steam-distilled and cold pressed can be added to vegetable oils, honey, yogurt, or fruit purees to make an edible addition to "all-consuming passion." Not recommended for absolute oils or the faint of heart.

Vata types, or people in Vata imbalance, need to relax, slow down, warm up, and become grounded into feeling their body, get out of their head, and be present in their sensuality, and for their partner. The use of angelica, clary sage, rose, saffron, lotus seed, jasmine, vanilla, geranium, ylang ylang, jatamansi (spikenard), patchouli, sandalwood, tuberose or champa will help create a sensual mood and build the hormonal and functional ability of the sex organs.

Pittas, or people in Pitta imbalance, need help letting go of anger and tension to feel their ecstatic nature. Grounding oils help, as do the cooling, calming nature of the flower oils. Pittas do best with angelica, champa, rose, chamomile, saffron, jasmine, geranium, ylang ylang, and sandalwood.

Kaphas, or people in Kapha imbalance, are slow to arouse and need stimulation to arouse hormones, "stimulate the juices," and dispel inertia and depression. Oils such as cinnamon, black pepper, clove, clary sage, yarrow, sage, aniseed, angelica, cypress, and rosemary are helpful.

133

Clove oil (as an anesthesia) can be used in a dilution of two drops per one-fourth ounce to de-sensitize the glands of the penis as an aid in preventing premature ejaculation or to enhance male ejaculatory control. Leave on until desired effect is achieved, then wipe off thoroughly or your partner will lose feeling too.

By enhancing all sensory experience during love-making (by including smells, food, sounds, feathers, massage, etc.) and prolonging the total experience, orgasm and ecstatic feeling can be moved from the genitals through the chakra system to other areas of the body. This is "Tantra": a world of expansive new experience. Margo Anand's *The Art of Sexual Ecstasy* is an excellent guide to this fascinating science, and essential oils can help set the mood.

CHAPTER FOURTEEN

COOKING WITH ESSENTIAL OILS

*I*t is important to remember that over fifty percent of all the essential oils produced today are used by the food flavoring industry. Essential oils are found in a majority of our prepared and preseasoned foods and are listed on the ingredients as "natural flavorings." Essential oils are preferred by the food and flavoring industry because once they are produced and placed in barrels, they will retain their strength, even getting stronger year by year, and they will not spoil. Dried herbs, however, lose their potency after a year, are subject to insect and rodent infestation, and take up to a hundred times more space. It is important to remember that one drop of essential oil is equal to one to two teaspoons of powdered herb.

Herbs were originally used in food not to increase flavor, but to increase digestion and preservation. The same can be said for essential oils, as many of the oils listed below are carminative, assist in the digestive process, and have antibacterial properties.

When cooking hot foods, such as soups, it is best to add the essential oils at the last possible moment in order to avoid losing the volatile essentials into the air.

Allspice may be used in desserts and puddings.

Angelica has been traditionally used in the making of liquor. A member of the celery family, it can be used in soups.

Anise has been traditionally used in liquors such as the Greek ouzo, and because of its ability to decongest and cool the liver, it would seem a particularly Ayurvedic way to drink alcohol. It can also be used to flavor desserts, in fruit leather, and in drinks, due to its licorice-associated taste.

Basil may be used in soups, pesto, spaghetti sauce and vegetable dishes. One to two drops per pint.

Bay may be used in soups, one drop per pint.

Cardamon is used traditionally in desserts, especially cookies, and coffee; one drop per cup of coffee or cup of flour.

Cinnamon may be added to cookies, pancakes, drinks, tea, or in yogurt lasse, one drop per pint.

Black pepper can be used on eggs, one drop per egg; in stews and soups, one drop per pint; salad dressings, one drop per cup.

Clove can be used in cakes, pies, cookies and teas.

Coriander for salad dressings, soups, desserts, beans and curries.

Cumin can be used with beans, curries, breads, salsas and peas.

Dhavana is used by Snapple® as a flavoring in some of its drinks. It has a strawberry aftertaste.

Dill finds special use in salad dressings, soups and stews.

Fennel for desserts and soups.

Ginger can be added to lemonade, drinks, teas, soups, curries and breads.

Grapefruit finds its use in drinks and pancakes.

Juniper may be used with vegetables, one drop per cup; also in fermenting sauerkraut or pickling vegetables.

Lavender is used extensively in France as a seasoning in soups and vegetables.

Lemon has use in drinks, desserts, ice creams, cakes, liquors, and pancakes.

Lemongrass is a favorite in Thai food, and for curries (especially coconut curry soup).

Marjoram may be added to soups, salads and dressings.

Nutmeg for desserts and lasses: equal parts of yogurt and water blended with seasonings and fruits.

Orange can be used in drinks, desserts, and pancakes.

Parsley for soups, breads, cheeses, and salad dressings.

Peppermint is especially good for desserts, cookies, drinks, and candies.

Rosemary for sauces, stews, poultry dishes.

Sage with poultry, salad dressings, soups, and sauces.

Tangerine can be used in drinks, desserts, and candies.

Thyme is especially good in soups and stew, and with vegetables.

Turmeric with curries, sauces, and vegetables.

Vanilla (oleo-resin), for candies, custards, pancakes and cakes.

CREATING A CHURNA (SEASONING MIXTURE) FOR THE DOSHAS

A churna is a mixture of seasonings blended to balance and support a specific dosha. It can be fun and easy once you have assembled the essential oils for your doshic type. You can use those steam-distilled and cold-pressed essential oils which are suitable as seasonings. Add one drop of your mixture to any food or drink you are consuming. Remember - avoid absolutes (essential oils extracted with petroleum solvents).

A **Vata** churna could include any of the following: angelica, mace, parsley, rose saffron, tarragon, vanilla, chamomile, cinnamon, clove, cumin, dill, fennel, ginger, lemongrass.

A **Pitta** churna can be composed of: chamomile, coriander, cumin, fennel, dill, lemon, lemongrass, lime, peppermint, rose, turmeric.

A **Kapha** churna can be made from any mix of angelica, anise, basil, bay, black pepper, cardamon, cinnamon, cloves, coriander, cumin, fennel, ginger, juniperberry. All spices are good for Kaphas; heating or cooling, they only add to the energetics and the prana.

MEDICATED GHEE

Ghee is also known as clarified butter. The process of making ghee removes the components of butter which have a tendency to go rancid or spoil, leaving behind a pure oil which is valued for its sattvic (harmonious) nature. Ghee will keep for long periods of time without refrigeration and can be used as an important vehicle for transporting the healing properties of herbs or oils into the skin or through your food into the GI tract.

Home Preparation of Ghee

Rather than buying expensive prepared products, it's always more empowering to make your own ghee, and its easy to make. In the West, convenience is everything, but ancient wisdom says the more involvement you have in your own healing or food preparation, the more beneficial that healing or that food will be for you. So the ghee you make yourself will have your personal energetics added to it, and will be much more helpful and healing to you than the ghee you buy. It is best to make ghee with unsalted butter, although the salt will, to a large extent, be removed if you do not have unsalted butter available.

In a large frying pan, slowly melt one pound of unsalted butter. Bring it to a light boil; a white foamy material will rise to the surface, which you can scoop off with a spoon or ladle and set aside. Continue to simmer and scoop for about fifteen minutes until the butter becomes clear. The foam can be discarded and what's left in the pan strained through a cheesecloth into a jar. As it cools, it will become more firm.

Medicated ghee is a tradition in India where various herbs (for specific purposes) are soaked in the liquid ghee for a month or more, after which the herbs are strained out, and the ghee used externally on the skin, or internally with food preparation. It's a big step for Westerner's to make their own ghee, and it may be a bit much to expect them to make medicated ghees with herbs. However, it only takes a few seconds to add essential oils to the fresh-made ghee to produce a medicated ghee with specific properties.

Recipe for Vata Ghee (for Digestion)

Add to ghee made from 1 lb. of butter as above: 2 drops ginger, 1 drop anise seed, 1 drop cardamon, 1 drop lemon

Recipe for Pitta Cooling Ghee

Add: 2 drops fennel, 2 drops coriander, 1 drop dill, 1 drop cardamon, 2 drops peppermint

Recipe for Kapha Energy-Moving Ghee

Add: 2 drops thyme, 2 drops juniper, 2 drops mint, 2 drops lemongrass, 1 drop ginger

These are just examples; any of the Vata-reducing essential oils, even the ones not customarily used in food, can be added to the ghee for medicinal effect.

CHAPTER FIFTEEN

THE HOME GODDESS

Ayurvedic Aromatherapy for Female Balance

THE EXPECTING MOTHER AND AYURVEDA

Giving birth is one of the most important experiences a woman can have. To go through the pregnancy and birth processes feeling clear, connected, devoted and loving, is to transfer those feelings to the child. To create this balance in mind and body, it can be helpful to treat pregnancy Ayurvedically.

Essential oils can be a great gift in relieving some of the symptoms of pregnancy, especially helpful for circulation and relaxation. Pregnancy is an opportunity to take care of yourself, to create transformation in your own life, and to prepare for birthing a soul waiting to experience the world. The more you work with your mind and emotions, the easier the birth. This is a period of creation, a time of contemplation, to help bring healing, not only to yourself but to the world. Some say that many of the spirits being born in these times are coming to prepare us for the healing of the planet. Others report that spirits of the Krishna lineage ("blue babies") are now incarnating onto the planet, especially to older, spiritually developed, women.

Everything that a woman experiences is directly transferred through her womb to the life inside. Massage, skin care, foot baths, compresses, inhalations, and bathing enhance a woman's pregnancy and increase the connectedness. Using an aroma lamp, spritzing and fragrancing the home can also be very beneficial. Remember to avoid excessive heat (sauna, hot baths) during pregnancy.

Pregnancy and Body Type

Vata: The Vata woman may have a tendency toward the following: back pain, groin pain, cramping, anxiety, fear, loss of weight (especially the first trimester), fatigue, insomnia, indigestion, bloatedness, excess gas, and varicose veins. The best oils for a Vata pregnancy: rosewood, chamomile, lavender, lemon, clary sage, vetiver, and ylang ylang.

Pitta: The Pitta pregnant woman will tend to have more frequent incidence of bladder infections, fever, irritation, anger, and fatigue. It can be aggravating to a Pitta to be in a process over which they have no control. Hemorrhoids and some hair loss are also common experiences. The essential oils most beneficial to a Pitta pregnancy are: lavender, rose, chamomile, sandalwood, clary sage, geranium, and jasmine.

Kapha: The Kapha pregnant woman will have a tendency to gain weight, experience water retention, fatigue, and lethargy, and crave sweets and starches. The most beneficial oils for a Kapha pregnancy are bergamot, clary sage, geranium, lavender, orange, jasmine, and rose.

All types may experience soreness of the breasts, morning sickness, and irritability.

Supporting Your Body During Pregnancy

Stretch Marks: Are small tears in the skin surface. At first you may see them as red or purplish marks which eventually fade to a lighter color than your skin. They are caused by rapid weight gain (you don't have to be pregnant to get them). You can assist the body in prevention by keeping the skin supple and elastic. Essential oils can help to minimize the scarring of the skin. Massage or oil your body with essential oil blends once a day, especially your stomach, breasts and thighs. The best oils for countering this condition are frankincense, tangerine, rose, chamomile, neroli, sage, rosewood, and geranium, diluted with the appropriate vegetable oils.

Relaxing Baths: To help drain away stress, center, and add joy to pregnancy:

Pitta: 5 drops chamomile, 2 drops tangerine, 3 drops lavender, 2 drops geranium.

Vata: 5 drops rosewood, 2 drops vetiver, 3 drops geranium, 2 drops clary sage.

Kapha: 5 drops orange, 5 drops cypress, 5 drops bergamot, 5 drops clary sage.

Massage: Once-a-week massage keeps the skin and body supple, relaxes the mind and prepares the muscles for birthing.

Pitta: to 2 ounces vegetable oil, add: 5 drops Roman chamomile, 2 drops rose, and 2 drops neroli.

Vata: to 2 ounces vegetable oil, add: 5 drops rosewood, 3 drops geranium, and 5 drops sandalwood.

Kapha: to 2 ounces vegetable oil, add: 5 drops orange, 2 drops bergamot, and 2 drops lavender.

For mixed types: Notice what dosha your symptoms correspond to and choose accordingly.

Nosebleed: Pitta women especially can experience this distressing symptom. Compress: 3 drops cypress and 2 drops lavender added to a cool, damp, wash cloth. Put over the nose area.

Toothache: Due to increased need for calcium, toothaches are more common during pregnancy.
    Add 1 drop blue chamomile or 1 drop clove to a wet cotton ball or on the end of a cotton swab. Apply to area of pain (tooth or gum).

Varicose Veins: to 2 ounces vegetable oil, add: 5 drops lavender, 5 drops geranium, 5 drops cypress, and 5 drops lemongrass; apply to affected area and massage veins twice a day.

Fluid Retention - Edema: (foot bath) 10 drops lavender, 3 drops cypress, 3 drops orange and 2 drops patchouli.

Poor Circulation: 5 drops rose, 5 drops clary sage, 5 drops cypress and 5 drops lavender in 2 ounces vegetable oil; massage into the skin.

Preparing for Childbirth (last 2 weeks): to 4-5 teaspoons vegetable oil, add: 3 drops nutmeg, 3 drops cloves, 2 drops sage, and 1 drop neroli; massage 2 to 3 drops on belly.

Oils to take to the hospital: rosewood, lavender, clary sage, bergamot and any oil you really like for diffusion, aroma lamp, massage, etc.

Oils to avoid during pregnancy: angelica, anise seed, basil, camphor, cedarwood, champa, citronella, hyssop, jasmine, juniper, lemon balm, lovage, marjoram, melissa, mustard, myrrh, pennyroyal, peppermint, rosemary, sage, savory, Spanish thyme, tarragon, thyme, and wintergreen.

POST-PARTUM CARE

Insufficient Engorgement: 2 drops geranium and 2 drops peppermint - apply to the breasts as a compress.

Cracked Nipples: 4 drops rose, 2 drops lemon and 2 tablespoons vegetable oil. Massage into irritated tissue.

Postpartum Depression: 3 drops neroli and 3 drops bergamot as an inhalation.

Painful Menstruation: (massage) to 2 tablespoons vegetable oil, add 5 drops chamomile, 5 drops lemon balm, 5 drops clary sage, and 2 drops ylang ylang.

Mastitis: Pitta-reducing diet and blue chamomile cool compresses.

BABY CARE

Teething: 3 drops chamomile, 3 drops yarrow, 3 drops lavender and 1 tablespoon vegetable oil.

Earache: 1 drop lavender, 1 drop cajeput, 1 tablespoon olive oil. Add 3 drops into the middle of a cotton ball, roll the cotton tightly, and place in ear. It is helpful to massage front and sides of the baby's neck with essential massage oil.

MENOPAUSE

Light: About three years ago (while Bryan and I were traveling and teaching), I began having some unusual and alarming symptoms with my menstrual period. My breasts became swollen and tender, and my period didn't come for three months. I thought that I might be pregnant and the idea of having a baby at 47 was not a turn-on for me or Bryan. I was especially alarmed because it has been a pattern for women in my family to have babies late in life. Just when I had finally accustomed myself to the idea of pregnancy, my period came with bleeding so severe I thought I might be miscarrying. The flushing (hot flashes) made me finally realize that I was experiencing symptoms of pre-menopause.

I called my mother for advice and asked her how menopause had been for her. She said that her culture did not even have a word for menopause, that only in the West was it regarded as a disease and attacked with synthetic hormones, drugs, painkillers, anti-depressants, muscle relaxants and amphetamines (all of which have many possible dangerous side effects). Her mother had prepared her for this period in her life by recommending special herbs and regular vaginal oil massage. She experienced no sudden symptoms or distressing changes and continued to experience a normal menstrual cycle until age 67. My mother speculated that, most likely, all the travel and stress had aggravated my Vata, and she suggested warming, heating emmenagogue and rejuvenative herbs. I began to increase my use of the female-hormone-stimulating essential oils in addition to a Vata-pacifying lifestyle and regimen.

My mother also expressed that this is a wonderful time for a woman to experience her feminine powers, a time to connect with the Divine Mother, and that this is a period in our life where we can do all the things that we've put off because we were raising children. She also said that this would be a time when I can recreate my relationship with my husband and make up for the time I had lost in my coupleness while raising a family. As difficult as it was on the road, I was able to alter my lifestyle to include regular yoga and meditation and get in my dosages of herbs and oils.

During my research into appropriate herbs and therapies for "the change," I discovered a wonderful book by one of my mentors, Susun S. Weed, *Menopausal Years: The Wise Woman Way.* Her book is an insightful presentation of many different treatment options for "the change." She is a gift to the planet and all the women who come in contact with her books. Using my knowledge of Ayurveda, *The Yoga of Herbs* and the information in Susun's book, I was able to expand and add new essential oils that were female-hormone-stimulating and grounding. From the herbs that Susun recommended, I was able to pick and choose the ones that would be best for my Vata nature.

Vata Menopause

Any time between the ages of 35 and 65, women can begin to experience "the change." Menopause affects each woman differently. Vata women will notice increased anxiety and nervousness, occasional anemia, leg cramps, headaches, irritability, dissatisfaction with their present relationships (sometimes leading to breakup), and irregular, scanty, periods. Yoni (vaginal) dryness, thinning of the vaginal tissues, cracked skin and nails, weight loss (especially in the arms and legs) and sometimes abdominal distention from constipation, are frequent symptoms. These can be countered by eating a

Vata-reducing diet, adopting a Vata-reducing lifestyle regimen, and regular exercise.

The following essential oils can speedily return balance to the Vata woman: angelica, with its immune-stimulating, grounding and tissue-building qualities, is known to reduce confusion; cedarwood (especially Himalayan cedarwood) is calming, relaxing, comforting, warming and stimulating to the mind. Clary sage has rejuvenative, aphrodisiac, antidepressant and female immune-stimulating qualities, while it builds tissue in the uterus and is excellent for relieving intestinal and uterine cramps. Dhavana decreases anxiety and fear, balances the female immune system, and is excellent for preventing cysts. The Ayurvedic College of Bombay is doing a ten-year study of women with uterine cancer using Dhavana, and the preliminary results are encouraging. Ginger has warming qualities, is grounding and calming, helps with dizziness, is strengthening, helps to increase energy levels, regulates moisture, and raises the body temperature. Carrot seed is very moisturizing to the tissue, and helps to create a glowing healthy skin. Jatamansi (spikenard) can be progesterone-stimulating, good for aging skin, and is grounding and relaxing. Rose helps with irregular menstruation, migraine headaches, detoxification of the liver, and encourages patience and love. Rosewood helps to relieve tiredness, nervousness, stress, and it is very grounding, giving you a sense of protection. The essential oil of seaweed is balancing and calming like the sea. It restores sexual interest and enjoyment, helps with joint pains, and is nourishing to the hair and skin. St. Johns wort essential oil is anti-inflammatory and can be helpful with joint pain. Valerian root is calming and sedating to the nervous system, but use caution; long term use of valerian root can create a dullness in the mind. Sandalwood helps with insomnia, anxiety, frigidity, and calms emotions. Vetiver is excellent for grounding, strengthening and nervousness. For dry yoni, we recommend Jeanne Rose's "Rose Cream," (see Resource Guide).

Pitta Menopause

When out of balance, the Pitta woman will experience anger, frustration, extreme hot flashes, loss of energy, loss of focus, frequent periods, severe flooding, extreme sweating, menopausal acne and even hair loss. The following essential oils would be most appropriate for Pitta imbalance: clary sage, balm (melissa) and rose will be effective at reducing anger, frustration, fevers and vaginitis; lemon balm, a hormone and blood pressure balancer, is also helpful with anger and excess sweating. Champa is an aphrodisiac, hormone balancer and mood enhancer; dhavana can be used for inflammations and yeast infections; lemon aids broken blood vessels and extreme bleeding with its astringency. Lemongrass is refreshing, aids concentration, and reduces varicose veins, lymph swelling or obstruction. Lavender is a balancer, is calming, sedative, helpful in mood swings, hair loss, acne and high blood pressure. Mint is refreshing, cooling, reduces mental fatigue, lack of concentration, acne and cramps. Myrtle counters acne, clarifies the mind, and is deodorizing; it can reduce the sour smells that sometimes come with hot flashes. Sandalwood assists uterine disorders, cystitis, and is harmonizing and tissue-regenerating. Yarrow is anti-inflammatory, regulates menstruation, helps in varicose veins, acne and amenohrrea (lack of period).

Kapha Menopause

Kapha women will have a tendency toward fluid retention, swelling, breast tenderness, fibroids, crying jags, loneliness and fatigue. They may want to sleep excessively, can feel unsupported, and become extremely sensitive. Essential oils to counter these symptoms include juniper for reducing swelling and excess fluids, cypress for fluid retention and to uplift the mind. Cypress allows the mind to collect itself and takes people out of sorrow and depression; it regulates female hormones and helps with ovarian cysts. Bay is a decongestant, balances the female endocrine system, the autonomic nervous system, and the circulatory system. Clary sage is antidepressant, revitalizing and aphrodisiac, and helps rejuvenate the female system. Sage detoxifies, heats up the body, cleanses and balances and stimulates perspiration, especially during hot flashes. It is a specific for water retention problems, depression, and hormonal imbalance. Geranium is immune-system stimulating, firms and tightens tissue and is mood elevating. Orange is uplifting for emotions, is warming and helpful in bladder and kidney disorders.

All of these essential oils can be added to your skin lotions, massage creams, shampoos, creme rinses, and baths. Many may be used internally in food, teas, douches and implants. For appropriate doses, consult Chapter Thirteen, "Personal Care," and Chapter Fourteen, "Cooking with Essential Oils."

Exercise

Kapha women should encourage perspiration by taking hot baths and engaging in aerobic exercise or dance. Pitta women should engage in swimming. Vata women can benefit from Tai Chi or Yoga.

Essential Oil Patch

To make an essential oil patch, soak a cotton ball or gauze in about ten drops of evening primrose oil or flaxseed oil, and add the essential oils of choice for your specific dosha and/or condition (up to three drops of each essential oil). Place the patches directly over the ovaries, just above the pubic bone, using adhesive tape to hold them against the skin. These patches can be freshened by adding more essential oil later in the day, or may be

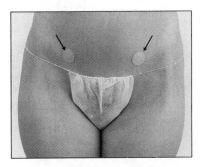

Essential Oil Patches

changed twice a day. For ease and convenience, regular or dot bandages, such as Band-Aids®, can be used instead of cotton or gauze.

The Ear Patch Story

Light: One of my students had a full hysterectomy and was on estrogen replacement therapy. She was sensitive to the adhesive on various types of tape, including Band-Aids®, and so she devised a small cotton crochet bag which she fills with cotton and places around the ear so the bag rests behind the lobe (almost like a hearing aid). She soaks the cotton with evening primrose oil and essential oils and wears it all the time. She has used this for one year, has not resorted to her estrogen replacement, and at a recent examination, her doctor found she was doing well and told her to keep up whatever she was doing. She has shared this method (and her recipe) with many women, all with encouraging results.

Ruth's Kapha Menopause Recipe

> 1/2 oz flax seed oil
> 1/2 oz almond oil
> 4 drops rose
> 12 drops ylang ylang
> 11 drops clary sage
> 11 drops yarrow

CHAPTER SIXTEEN

HEALTH ENHANCEMENT

IMMUNE DISORDERS

ALLERGIES

Allergies are a symptom of a body out of balance, an immune system depressed, possible toxic build-up and poor digestion. Ayurveda would first cleanse the channels (pancha karma), balance the doshas (diet-lifestyle), build up the immune system (rasayana) and increase the efficiency of the digestion.

It is helpful to determine which foods are bothering you, to keep a record of those foods (see Diet-Symptom Diary on following page), avoid them for a period, then rotate them into your diet, i.e., once every four to seven days. Those essential oils which assist digestion and immune response, clear channels, and balance dosha imbalance will assist with allergy problems.

The following oils can be especially helpful with allergies and may be used in all the possible ways. Inhalations and diffusers will help most with nasal and respiratory allergies; essential oil baths, lotions and massage oils with skin allergies; and food-drink flavoring with gastro-intestinal tract symptoms.

Vata: immortelle, gold, chamomile, lavender, angelica, clary sage

Pitta: lavender, lemongrass, lemon balm, labdanum, myrtle, rose, blue chamomile

Kapha: eucalyptus, elecampane, patchouli, hyssop, myrtle

151

DIET-SUMMARY DIARY

NOTE: this page can be photocopied.

Name _____   Date _____

Page of Diary _____

INSTRUCTIONS:

Take your pulse in the morning upon awakening.
Take your pulse before and after every meal.
Write down when and what you eat and how you feel.
Write down any reactions; physical, mental, emotional or spiritual.

Example:

Time	Morning Pulse		
7:45 am	High Vata		

Time	Food and Drinks Consumed	Pulse	Symptoms
8:00 am	Eggs, Toast, Bacon, Coffee	Vata->Pitta	Fullness
9:00 am			Headache, indigestion

Time   Morning Pulse

_____

Time   Food and Drinks Consumed   Pulse   Symptoms

ARTHRITIS

The opening of this book describes three patients, each with a different type of arthritis, receiving three different prescriptions from an Ayurvedic physician, determined by their body types. Here is a more detailed explanation of how each type of arthritis develops and is corrected.

Vata arthritis begins with an accumulation of excess Vata and overflow from the colon into the circulation, settling eventually in the joints, accompanied by ama. The auto-immune system then attacks the joint surfaces, creating pain, dryness, stiffness, and cracking. In addition to traditional Vata-reducing therapies, moist heat in the form of hot baths and, particularly, hot castor oil or sesame oil compresses, combined with essential oils such as camphor, cinnamon, calamus, eucalyptus, valerian, rosemary, angelica, and blue chamomile, can provide relief. A very strong massage oil can be used to oil the entire body, with special attention on the joints. It is recommended that dairy products and foods in the nightshade family, i.e., potato, eggplant, etc., be eliminated as an additional precaution. If heat increases the pain, suspect Pitta-variety arthritis.

Pitta arthritis is characterized by heat, swelling and burning. It begins when excess Pitta and the acid by-products of metabolism overflow from the small intestine, migrate through circulation, and settle in the joints. In addition to general Pitta reduction methods, use cool compresses and coconut oil liniment with the following Pitta-reducing essential oils: calendula, chamomile, lemon balm, turmeric, sandalwood and benzoin. Sweet dairy products may have to be taken off the Pitta-reducing diet. If cool compresses increase pain, you might be dealing with Kapha or Vata forms of arthritis.

Kapha arthritis begins when Kapha builds up in excess in the lungs and sinuses, slowing digestion and metabolism, and blocking the elimination of ama. In some individuals the joints become congested, swollen, loose, with dull aching. These symptoms can be relieved by hot baths, compresses and massage with mustard oil, using the following essential oils: rosemary, juniper, basil, mugwort, orange, cinnamon, camphor, cypress. Dry heat (dry sauna) or a heating pad is also effective. Suspect Pitta arthritis if heat aggravates the condition.

External measures are helpful in all three types of arthritis, but elimination of ama and reduction of excess doshas through pancha karma and general measures, is vital for any lasting reversal of the condition.

THE COMMON COLD

Western medicine offers little that is effective against viruses (the common cold, influenza, etc.) except to manage symptoms. Often the products used are counter to the immune response of the body. For instance, when a cold virus is attempting to establish colonies in the nasal mucosa, the sinuses instinctively discharge a steady stream of mucous to carry the virus away— out of the nose or down the throat to the stomach, where hydrochloric acid will kill it. Antihistamines can dry the membranes, preventing the body's vital defense tactic.

Fever is the body's way to raise the metabolic rate, increasing the movement of white blood cells, and raising the body's temperature out of the preferred range of the pathogens. Yet if we take aspirin or Tylenol® to lower fever, we defeat the body's natural responses.

Many essential oils have strong anti-viral properties and can assist the body in overcoming a cold. Inhalation, nose drops, gargles, "vapor rubs," room diffusion, baths, and internal use in drinks (not food) are all recommended.

Vata: ginger, camphor, cinnamon, anise, lemon, rosewood, angelica, basil, eucalyptus, cajeput

Pitta: chamomile, coriander, lime, peppermint, sandalwood, yarrow

Kapha: basil, clove, eucalyptus, niaouli, hyssop, rosemary, sage, savory

HERPES
(cold sores, fever blisters and genital)

Dr. David Frawley, in *Ayurvedic Healing,* gives an excellent description of the Ayurvedic approach to herpes.

Vata: Lesions are dry, hard, and painful. Pain is alleviated by the use of bergamot, trifolia, tea tree, lemon, niaouli, gold chamomile, and geranium.

Pitta: Lesions will be hot, red and swollen. Internal and external use of cooling essential oils can assist in treatment. Oils include: lavender, neem, blue chamomile, rock rose, tea tree, yarrow, and rosewood.

Kapha: Lesions exhibit a clear-to-whitish discharge and are not particularly red or painful. The patient is helped by cajeput, tea tree, sage, eucalyptus, lemon, and niaouli.

A beeswax salve can be helpful in exterior lesions of all types.

KIDNEY AND BLADDER INFECTIONS

Infections are most often a high Pitta condition and are characterized by burning and painful urination with blood or pus, yellow to red in color. When Vata is involved, the urination will be scanty, irregular, and painful, sometimes accompanied by back and flank pain. Kapha involvement is characterized by dull pain, heaviness, and mucous discharge.

Internal use may alleviate symptoms; one to three drops three times a day of the following diuretic oils in drink or food. External use of compresses can be helpful (warm for Vata and Kapha, cool for Pitta).

Vata: lemon, rock rose, Himalayan cedar, cedarwood, benzoin, lemongrass, sandalwood, and sweet orange

Pitta: lemongrass, spearmint, fennel, coriander, niaouli, sandalwood, lavender, tea tree, yarrow, chamomile

Kapha: juniperberry, cubeb, cinnamon, parsley, orange, eucalyptus, myrtle, cajeput, basil, hyssop, cypress

Urinary tract infections are more difficult to treat if the patient's urine is alkaline, because bacteria prefer an alkaline environment. Acidifying the urine with ascorbic acid "C" (not ascorbate), and consuming berries such as cranberry, blueberry, etc., can make a difference. The berries contain pigments which coat the urinary tract, making it slippery and difficult for the pathogens to establish colonies.

COMMON ILLNESS

GASTRO-INTESTINAL SYSTEM

Stomach Complaints

Stomach and digestive problems are one of the most common complaints of Western man, as witnessed by all the media advertising for anti-acids and laxatives. Much difficulty could be avoided by taking time to "really" bless our food, by eating slowly with no distractions (except congenial conversation), thoroughly masticating (chewing) every bite, drinking only minimally during or after the meal, and not overeating.

In addition to the thoughtful addition of oils to food or tea, they can be used externally in a tummy rub, compress, or inhalation.

Vata's excitability and nervous nature carries over into digestion, and they can suffer gas, bloating, cramps, and pain. These conditions can be relieved by using the following essential oils: angelica, anise, bay, cardamon, chamomile, fennel, ginger, tarragon, valerian, and other carminatives.

Pitta's fiery nature reflects in burning, ulcers, fast digestion, constant hunger, and gastritis, and is relieved by using chamomile, clary sage, coriander, cumin, fennel, dill, lemon balm, lime, mint, saffron and yarrow.

Kapha's gentle, watery character sometimes shows up as slow digestion, mucous accumulation, loss of taste, and weight gain. All carminatives, but especially heating and stimulating essential oils, will remedy the imbalance, including: clove, bay, cardamon, ginger, juniper, oregano, parsley, and thyme.

Ulcers

In **Vata** excess, ulcers can be caused by too much dry, cold food, hot spices, irregular eating habits, fear and worry; and are characterized by pain and insufficient mucous protection. Warm compresses of anise, lemon, and gold chamomile are advisable in addition to traditional measures.

Pitta ulcers may be produced by an aggressive nature and too much hot spice, causing excess hydrochloric acid and burning. Cool compresses of benzoin, blue chamomile, lavender, mints, and fennel can soothe the symptoms.

Kaphas have ulcers less commonly, but may be associated with slow digestion, grief, attachment, nausea and dull pain. Warm compresses of myrrh and cumin and the use of carminative herbs are recommended.

> *Bryan:* I love essential oils, but if I ever manifested an ulcer I would drink three ounces of cabbage juice four times a day. It stops burning instantly and contains vitamin U, which helps repair ulcers.

Liver Disturbances

The liver is the chemical factory of the body and runs Pitta-hot (109 degrees Fahrenheit). It helps us emulsify fats for digestion (bile), breaks down and recycles the old tired red blood cells, stores sugar as glycogen for future energy needs, and hundreds of other lipid, protein, and enzyme functions.

Excess **Vata** reduces and dries up bile production, making fat and oil digestion difficult; interferes with blood sugar metabolism; lowers the liver heat, and causes light-colored, hard, bowel movements. Essential oils which stimulate liver activity include: labdanum, vetiver, rosemary, ginger, and turmeric.

Pitta excess causes inflammation, excess bile, diarrhea, (and anger) which can be eased with rose, lemon balm, mint, coriander, carrot seed oil, fennel, lavender, aloe vera, yarrow, and chamomile.

Kapha slowness and congestion can result in stasis, swelling, and congestion, which can be energetically assisted by rosemary, rose, cumin, basil, ginger, clove, caraway, black pepper, cajeput, and juniper. Use as compress or add to food and drink.

Gall Bladder

The gall bladder is the storing and regulating organ for the liver's bile. Western diet often predisposes toward cholesterol stones which can be reduced or eliminated by dietary changes, natural therapeutics (i.e., gall bladder flush - see following recipe), and ingesting lecithin, which emulsifies cholesterol anywhere in the body. Gall bladder congestion-obstruction is characterized by nausea upon eating rich foods, and upper back, right shoulder and right upper abdomen pain or sensitivity. The essential oils listed above for the liver also will assist in clearing the gall bladder.

In addition to the judicious (one to two drops) use of essential oil in food, compresses (hot for Vata-Kapha - cold for Pitta) over the lower right rib cage, or application of massage oil mixtures, are effective.

Recipe for Gall Bladder Flush

1. Fast for three days drinking 8 oz. apple juice every 2 hours, and taking 2 "oo" capsules of barberry bark every 4 hours (while awake). Go to sleep.

2. Perform an enema on the third night of the fast. Drink 4 oz. virgin olive oil and 4 oz. lemon juice. Go to sleep.

3. Small, green stones in an oily bowel movement may pass the following morning.

Pancreatic Disorders

The pancreas is actually two organs. The "tail" portion is an endocrine gland which produces insulin, and the "body" portion produces enzymes to digest protein, fats, and starches. It also produces bicarbonate (an alkaline substance) which is secreted into the digestive tract when food passes by. Bicarbonate reduces the high acidity of the food as it leaves the stomach, allowing the pancreatic enzymes to work. Pancreatic enzymes are not able to perform in an acid environment.

Excess **Vata** will dry up pancreatic secretions and cause indigestion and gas. Carminative (digestive) oils which will stimulate secretion include allspice, anise, bay, caraway, gold chamomile, cinnamon, cloves, cumin, dill, garlic, ginger, oregano, savory, tarragon and thyme. Use small amounts of oil (one to two drops) with food or drink, in a hot compress, or massage oil tummy rub.

Because of its hormone and enzyme production, the pancreas is governed by **Pitta**, but excess secretion can deplete the organ and cause burning and diarrhea. Cooling carminatives such as blue chamomile, coriander, cumin, fennel, dill, lemon balm, lavender, saffron, and mint with food, drink, or as a cool compress or tummy rub will calm pancreatic excess.

Kapha can have a sluggish pancreas and can be assisted by the prana (energy addition) of both lists of oils above.

Intestinal Disorders

Small Intestine

The small intestine is the most important organ for the absorption of nutrients. Vata obstruction, lack of secretions, or dryness, can affect this organ, and be assisted with Vata-reducing carminatives. Pitta- and Kapha-reducing carminatives are appropriate for the small intestine when those dosha excesses occur. Being the seat of Pitta, burning hot diarrhea can be indicative of excess Pitta in the small intestine.

Large Intestine

The large intestine is mainly responsible for absorbing moisture. Friendly bacteria such as acidophilus or bifidus keep bad bacteria and yeast away, help form the stool, and break down undigested food into nutrients for us to absorb.

Constipation

Many practitioners feel that constipation is the primary cause for many diseases common to Western people, including arthritis, immune disorders, and nervous system diseases.

Vata constipation is the most common and difficult to treat because the colon is the primary seat and overflow site for Vata. When Vata is obstructed, the ingestion of medicated ghee, castor or sesame oil (easy with essential oils) prepares and softens the GI tract. Medicated basti (enema) with oil retention follows; see page 202. Appropriate oils include ginger, anise, trifolia, gold chamomile, and basil. Warm compresses and abdominal massage can be soothing. Complete pancha karma cleansing and opening of all channels will prepare the patient for Vata-reducing therapies which will add substance and build tissue. Without first cleansing, rich food and herbs would only add to the undigested, uneliminated waste, and create more blockage.

Pitta types typically exhibit frequent and loose, oily stools and, if constipation occurs, mild laxatives, aloe vera, abdominal massage with trifolia and increased use of essential oils of immortelle, peppermint, lemongrass, chamomile, fennel, coriander, and mandarin will alleviate.

Kapha metabolism usually produces large, moist, well-formed stools once a day, but under stress they can slow down. Stronger laxatives are often needed (consult *Ayurvedic Healing* or *Yoga of Herbs*). Massage and compresses of black pepper, juniper, ginger, trifolia, and rosemary can be helpful.

Ingestion of medicated ghee made with the above oils would also be effective. Jeanne Rose, in *The Aromatherapy Book*, relates how just the smell of cumin oil was laxative for her baby.

Hemorrhoids

A common problem in the West, hemorrhoids are caused by constipation, straining, poor nutrition, and liver congestion, which can be corrected by the addition of fiber to the diet, astringent herbs, addition of vitamins C, E, B-complex, and bioflavinoids, and certain pigments from berries such as blueberries, raspberries, etc., which strengthen the walls of the blood vessel.

Vata hemorrhoids are painful and dry, with cracking. Pitta hemorrhoids burn, with much bleeding, and Kapha will be swollen with dull aching.

The following essential oils can be applied as a compress, in a vegetable oil retention enema, to a sitz bath (warm or cool water in a large bowl that you sit in for ten minutes at a time) or may be taken internally, two drops four times a day with food or drinks.

Pitta: clary sage, geranium, sandalwood, neroli, yarrow, myrtle

Vata: bergamot, valerian, patchouli, cypress, frankincense

Kapha: cajeput, myrrh, niaouli, cypress

CANDIDIASIS

Candidiasis is not just a female problem, but can become a systemic problem for anyone with lowered resistance, on steroids such as cortisone, estrogen or birth control, antibiotics, or anyone eating a diet high in sugars. The colon can be a problem area for these people. Yeast-fighting essential oils can help restore balance without disturbing friendly bacteria.

Vata: trifolia, gold chamomile, cinnamon bark, brahmi, rosewood and grapefruit

Pitta: tagetes, tea tree, blue chamomile, yarrow

Kapha: rosemary, eucalyptus, thyme, sage, and cajeput

Best administered with oil retention enemas (see enema-basti, page 202), or one to two drops added to food three times a day.

Oral Thrush is a form of candidiasis that manifests as white spots on swollen tonsils and can be assisted with a gargle made with the above essential oils in a ratio of two to four drops of oil to one cup of water. Agitate the mixture well, and use frequently throughout the day. You may swallow or spit out after use.

ESSENTIAL OILS AND THE ENDOCRINE ORGANS

Below are listed organs of the body and the essential oils which can be helpful in their function. Behind each essential oil is the letter V, P, or K, indicating that the oil assists those dosha types or imbalances.

Brain: brahmi (VPK); basil (VK), rosemary (VK), clary sage (VPK), jasmine (VK), ylang ylang (PK), sandalwood (VPK)

Pituitary: sage (K), clary sage (VPK), jasmine (VP), yarrow (PK), patchouli (VPK), ylang ylang (VP)

Pineal Gland: shamama (VPK), hina (VPK), sandalwood (VPK), sage (VK), champa (PK), rose (VPK)

Thyroid: seaweed absolute (VK) - (compress, external use), garlic (VK), parsley (VK), ajwan (celery seed oil) (VK)

Parathyroid: juniper (VIP), cypress (VK), seaweed absolute (VK)

Thymus Gland: eucalyptus (VK), lemon (VPK), camphor (PK), rosemary (PK), lemon balm (PK), thyme (K), angelica (VK)

Adrenals: thyme (VK), geranium (VP), lemon (VK), savory (VK), blue chamomile (VK), Moroccan chamomile (VPK), yarrow (PK), ylang ylang (PK), rosemary (VK)

Pancreas: eucalyptus (VK), black pepper (VK), fennel (VPK), ginger (VK), carrot seed (VK)

Ovaries: jatamansi (VK), jasmine (VPK), angelica (VK), dhavana (VK), clary sage (VPK), laudanum (VP), yarrow (PK)

Testes: jatamansi (VK), sage (VK), lemon (VPK), parsley (PK), savory (K)

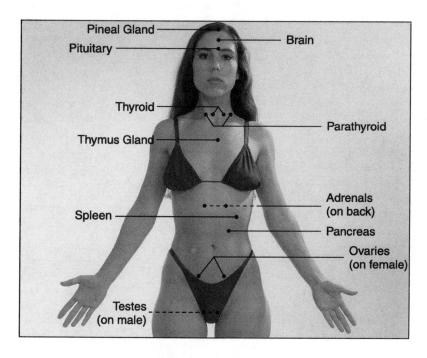

Locations of the Endocrine Organs

MIND, EMOTIONS AND SPIRIT

The seers say that we incarnate into this world with everything we have learned in our previous lives. Unless we are highly realized beings, we incarnate and forget all that we are. Our purpose in life and our needed experiences are incorporated into our karmic sheath in energetic form; this is why we are attracted to certain types of people, professions, situations, etc. The seers teach that we chose all of this before we came in: our parents, our body types and our experiences. Much of this happens without much awareness on our part. But once we reach the understanding that our ultimate purpose is to "know and serve," we are attracted to create the appropriate form of doing just that. We begin to achieve some degree of self mastery. Until that point we find ourselves locked into automatic responses dictated to us by our ego-mind from past experience. During this lifetime, events occur and we make judgments about what they mean: Every situation is compared to a similar past event, and projections are brought forward and applied to the new situation. Our ego-mind is a judging and evaluating machine.

THREE STATES OF MIND

Our mind is a filter through which all experience is passed. Each of us creates, inside our head, a world in which we live. Our ego-mind attempts to protect us from harm by keeping us separate; some doctors say the only disease is separation. Every moment we choose between heaven and hell (joining or separation) and the ego-mind will always choose safety and separation over vulnerability and openness.

Tamas

Ayurveda says there are three states of the mind in which we can play out our life experience. The first is dominated by darkness and dullness and is known as tamas. The Vata aspect of tamasic ego-mind is characterized by fearfulness, dishonesty, secretiveness, depression, self-destruction, addiction, perversion, and suicidal tendencies. The Pitta aspect of tamasic ego-mind is characterized by hate, vindictiveness outward destruction, and criminality. The Kapha aspect of tamas is characterized by dullness, lethargy, apathy, and insensitivity.

Rajas

Ayurveda teaches that when a person rises above darkness, he comes into the world of action. Rajas is being caught up in the illusion of the world and the pursuit of desires. For the Vata ego-mind in a rajasic state, your life will be full of indecisiveness, hyperactivity, irritation, anxiety, superficial conversations, noise and disruption. The Pitta rajasic mind is often angry, proud, critical, dominating, ambitious, impulsive and manipulative. Kapha mind in the rajasic state will manifest issues of control, attachment, greed, materialism, the pursuit of comfort, security, and sentimentality. Each of these modes of action, thoughts, and emotions contains lessons, and we cannot label them as good or bad. A human being can learn from anything, but in the illusion we become lost, thinking "this is all there is." But the seeker of light will find a higher source.

Sattva

Ayurveda says that sattva is the highest state, that this is our birthright, this is where we are meant to play and live. The Vata sattvic mind has the ability to make positive changes, to start projects, to have enthusiasm and under-standing of human connectedness, quick comprehension, good communica-tion, flexibility, energy and a strong healing force. The Pitta mental nature makes a good leader who is clear, enlightened, discriminating, intelligent, warm, friendly and independent. The Kapha personality type manifests sattvic qualities and is notably calm, stable, loyal, peaceful, compassion-ate, devoted, nurturing and receptive.

BREAKING OLD EMOTIONAL PATTERNS

What we have done in the past is not important, except as fuel for growth. It is said that "he who knows not history, is doomed to repeat it." Our personal histories are most important for us to know, so that we don't find ourselves caught in patterns of behavior which take us nowhere. Essential oils can be the key in breaking that cycle. Our sense of smell is strongly connected into our limbic system, our moods, our memories, our desires, our appetites. Below please find a list of emotions and some suggested essential oils that you can use in inhalations, personal perfumes, diffusers, spritzers, and baths, to help to break your patterns.

Essential Oils to Bring the Vata Ego-Mind to the Sattvic State

Fearful, anxious:
Angelica, cypress, jatamansi, Himalayan cedarwood, clary sage, cyperus, benzoin, rosewood, bergamot, frankincense, geranium, jasmine, lavender, lemongrass, orange, sandalwood, vanilla, vetiver and ylang ylang.

Scattered, feeling ungrounded:
Angelica, eucalyptus, sandalwood, vetiver, spikenard, chamomile.

Weak:

Angelica, trifolia, basil, cardamon, rosemary.

Moody:

Benzoin, bergamot, clary sage, elemi, frankincense, geranium, rosewood.

Unfocused:

Basil, cypress, lemon, lemongrass, rose, rosemary, petitgrain.

Absentminded:

Basil, cypress, lemon, orange, rosemary.

Sleepless (insomnia):

Basil, chamomile, lavender, mandarin, orange, neroli, rose, rosemary, thyme.

Essential Oils to bring Pitta Ego-Mind to the Sattvic State

Angry:

Borage, cardamon, champa, coriander, blue chamomile, lotus, musk, rose, saffron.

Stubborn:

Lavender and peppermint.

Opinionated:

Jasmine and yarrow.

Hurtful:

Hina, oud musk, geranium and yarrow.

Domineering:

Amber and geranium.

Frustrated:

Brahmi and gold chamomile.

Irritable:
Benzoin, frankincense, lavender, Roman chamomile, rose, ylang ylang.

Essential Oils to bring Kapha Ego-Mind to the Sattvic State

Depressed:
Bergamot, lemongrass, geranium, clary sage, grapefruit, orange, petitgrain.

Disinterested:
Lavender, champa, orange, bergamot, cajeput, patchouli.

Greedy:
Basil, rosemary, cardamon.

Attached:
Mint, ginger, myrtle.

Uncertain (low self-esteem):
Ylang ylang, immortelle, petitgrain, jasmine.

Resistant:
Grapefruit, lime, bergamot, chamomile.

Sad:
Benzoin, jasmine, rose, rosewood, clary sage, melissa, neroli.

CHAPTER EIGHTEEN

INDIAN MASSAGE AND MARMA POINT THERAPY

Light: As a child, our family traveled all over the world. Some of my deepest memories are of returning to my grandmother's house; the long evenings we spent together, the whole family massaging each other (unlike the West, where everyone watches television). Grandmother had an herb garden and a whole cabinet full of medicated oils that she made seasonally. She also had an extensive collection of essential oils from India. My mother always brought her new oils from wherever we had traveled.

In India, it is the custom for a mother and baby to be massaged every day for forty days after the birth. The child continues to be massaged daily until the age of three. The practice of baby massage is beautifully explained and pictorially demonstrated in Frederick LeBoyer's book, *With Loving Hands.* Often when traveling through India, even in the open marketplace, you will see mothers with their blankets spread on the ground, with their babies reclined on their straightened legs, giving massage.

Because we traveled in many countries and observed many customs, my mother always needed to remind me to go and sit at my grandfather's feet when we first got to his house; to show my respect and love for him by giving him a foot massage. In family gatherings, it was a custom that the men would talk, and the women would all go somewhere and do massage.

171

While in school at UC Berkeley, I became aware of how stressed everyone was, especially during finals; and how people never touched one another. I began to massage my friends, and pretty soon my room became "the place" to come and relax and get rid of tension. This was the first time I realized that massage could be a profession.

Later when I traveled through Mexico and Central America with two Swamis (Swami Tilak and Swami Jyoti), I massaged their feet and they taught me systematic Marma points. They were my first real teachers in Ayurveda.

SPECIFIC MASSAGE OILS FOR DOSHA IMBALANCE

When practicing Indian massage, it is important to use a massage oil/essential oil combination appropriate for lowering the imbalanced dosha. You can determine this mixture by having your patient take the questionnaire beginning on page 24 to determine their body type and imbalance. Another alternative would be to have them take the subdosha symptom survey (pages 50-52) to determine which of the subdoshas are the most out of balance.

When an individual is badly out of balance, essential oil massage should be done at least three times a week. As they come back into balance, once a week is a marvelous gift that we all should give ourselves, with self-massage part of a daily regimen.

Massage Oils for Vata

All oils are good for Vata, especially sesame and hazelnut oil used in combination with any of the Vata-reducing essential oils found on page 94, but especially angelica, basil, calamus, camphor, cardamon, chamomile, clary sage, coriander, eucalyptus, ginger, lavender, lemongrass, sandalwood, vetiver and jatamansi (spikenard). Mix the essential oils into vegetable oil at a ratio of approximately 50 drops essential oil to four ounces of vegetable oil.

Massage Oils for Pitta

Essential oils for Pitta are best mixed with cooling oils such as olive and coconut, and would include Pitta-reducing oils (found on page 99) especially chamomile, coriander, cumin, fennel, jasmine, jatamansi, lemon balm, lemongrass, lavender, peppermint, rose, sandalwood, spearmint, vetiver and yarrow. Mix the essential oils into the vegetable oil at a ratio of approximately 50 drops essential oil to four ounces of vegetable oil.

Massage Oils for Kapha

Kaphas are best treated with heating vegetable oils such as almond, mustard and canola, although Ayurvedically, Kaphas do less well with oils in general, and often, massage is done with alcohol, powders or silk gloves to avoid adding too much oil to the Kapha metabolism. Essential oils which are effective for Kapha would include angelica, basil, camphor, cardamon, cinnamon, eucalyptus, ginger, myrrh, orange peel, sage, and yarrow, and other oils found on page 103. Mix the essential oils into the vegetable oil at a ratio of approximately 75-100 drops to four ounces of vegetable oil.

DIFFERENT STROKES FOR DIFFERENT FOLKS
Massage According to Dosha Type

Each dosha type requires a different type of massage according to the qualities which are exhibited by the dosha imbalance.

Vata Massage

Because Vatas are already dry, cold, irregular, and rough, they need to have a massage which is oily, warm, smooth and nurturing. Stroking should be firm, but smooth. Abrupt, rough movements can be irritable and disturbing to Vata types. Lots and lots of warm oil should be used. Excess oil can be allowed to sit on the skin (after you've worked on the area) to soak in; Vata bodies will just absorb it. Oil should be allowed to stand and soak into the tissue over the entire abdomen. Keep Vatas warm with sheets, heating pads, even blankets.

Pitta Massage

Pittas are oily, hot, intense and fluid, so they need a massage which is calming and relaxing. They do not need as much oil as Vata types and their oils need to be of a cooling nature. The massage should be deep and varied, and the subject's mind can be kept occupied by using different techniques. Pitta tissues can sometimes be inflamed or irritated, so care should be used in these areas. Too much fast movement can worsen their imbalance; the massage needs to be slow and deliberate without a lot of movement from one area to another. Pittas can become irritable if the therapist is not centered.

Kapha Massage

Kaphas require the most vigorous type of massage to stimulate their sluggish metabolism and lack of fluid movement. Fast, even harsh, movements are appropriate, with as little oil as possible. If the Kapha is really out of balance, increasing amounts of diaphoretic and diuretic essential oils will be helpful. Since you will be using less oil, you can increase the mixture to approximately 75-100 drops of essential oil to four ounces of vegetable oil. During the massage, it's important to draw Kaphas into conversation so they can explore and let go of their own feelings, which they are usually reticent to divulge.

MARMA POINTS AND ESSENTIAL OILS

Marma points are energy centers of the body. Marma means secret, hidden and vital. The Chinese used marma points to develop the complex system of energy points known as the acupuncture meridian system. These points were used in ancient times to energetically harm the enemy by wounding or striking a blow at these vital spots. Physicians also studied these points in order to heal soldiers wounded in battle.

Marma points are points of connection between the physical body and the subtle energetic bodies. They often relate to specific muscles, organs or tissues. Marma points can be used in self massage or massaging others in order to balance energies, restore normal function, energize or relax. Marma points are traditionally used in combination with Indian massage but can be used alone or with other methods.

Marma points are located on the body by taking finger measurements from various points. Because people have different size fingers, the patient's own fingers are used to measure. Marma points are not as specific as acupuncture points, and in fact, can be as large as six inches across. For the purposes of this book, we have used a chart and written descriptions to help locate the points.

Traditionally, medicated oils were used to energize and massage these marma points. Here in the West, essential oils have been substituted as they are much more common and are in fact stronger and more potent than medicated oils. Because each marma point refers to an anatomical area or body function, specific essential oils will appropriately stimulate that part or function. In listing the marma points, we will give their number (our system), their Indian name, location, the body part or function to which they refer, and a few of the many essential oils associated with their stimulation.

Marma points are massaged with the thumb. A drop of warm oil is applied to the marma point before massage; this oil will be premixed with the appropriate vegetable and essential oils for the individual and the condition being treated. Start with small, gentle, clockwise circles, moving outward and then back inward, slowly increasing pressure, outward, inward, in ever increasing and decreasing circles. Perform about five circles going out and five circles coming back: do this three times. Marma points which are blocked or out of balance will be more tender and painful than other marma points. If you suspect a marma point is blocked, you may add one drop of a specific essential oil for that marma point, right onto the area where you have already applied the general massage oil. This additional stimulation will energetically free up the point.

MARMA POINTS

Indian Name	Location	Function/area of Body Affected	Essential Oils	
Arm				
1a. Kshipra	Base of Thumb	Passion Connection to Will Stomach	Cardamon Sandalwood	Fennel Carminatives
b. Kshipra	Base of Little Finger	Passion Connection to Will Stomach	Cardamon Sandalwood	Fennel Carminatives
2a. Talhridaya	Center of Palm	Heart	Cardamon Rose	Orange
b. Talhridaya	Tips of Fingers	Nervousness Circulation	Sandalwood Champa	Rosewood Ylang Ylang
3. Manibandha	Thumb Side of Wrist	Expressing Yourself in the World	Vetiver Rosewood	Jatamansi Valerian
4. Koorchsha	Little Finger Side of Wrist	Circulation	Lavender Juniper Orange	Cypress Keawa
5. Karpooram	Middle Front of Elbow	Sexual Metabolism	Cinnamon Jatamansi	Clove Dhavana
6. Kurpara	Inside and Outside of Elbow	Right—Liver, Gallbladder Left—Spleen	Ginger Myrtle	Rose Rosemary Coriander
7. Oorvi	Outer, Middle Arm	Blood Circulation	Thyme Camphor Clove	Eucalyptus Orange
Neck				
8. Kraknrik	One Inch Below Base of Skull to Side of Spine	Heart Opening Lungs Chest Congestion	Cajeput Eucalyptus	Basil
9. Unnamed	Center Base of Skull	Mental Fatigue Allergies	Rosemary Basil Myrtle	Lemongrass All Citrus
10. Manya	Front of Neck Under Ear	Blood Vessels Circulation	Rosemary Lavender	Juniper Geranium
11. Siramantrika	Lower Front of Neck	Mother of All Vessels	Myrtle Camphor Cypress	Eucalyptus Sandalwood Cajeput

Indian Name	Location	Function/area of Body Affected	Essential Oils	
Chest				
12. Neela	Chestbone/ Collarbone Junction	Thyroid 5th Chakra	Seaweed Absolute	Cajeput Sandalwood
13. Apastamgh	Right Upper Chest Below Collar Bone	Muscle Tone Heart	Rosemary Cardamon	Lemongrass Rose
14. Kakshadhara	Left Upper Chest Below Collar Bone	Muscle Tone Heart	Rosemary Cardamon	Lemongrass Rose
15a. Hridayam	Upper Central Chest	Thymus 4th Chakra	Yarrow Saffron Myrtle	Cumin Angelica Rose
b. Hridayam	Lower Central Chest	Heart	Cardamon Saffron	Rose Orange
16. Manipura	Lower Tip of Sternum	3rd Chakra Will	Sandalwood Dhavana	Anise/ Champa
Abdomen				
17. Nabi	2" Below Navel	Balance Creativity Elimination 2nd Chakra	Ginger Trifolia Cedarwood	Clary Sage Cypress
18. Vasth	On Central Pubic Bone	Sexual Energy Survival	Ginger Dhavana Sandalwood	Yarrow Trifolia
Leg (front)				
19. Lohitaksham	Groin-Inguinal Ligament	Lymph Drainage	Rose Nutmeg Ylang Ylang	Geranium Jasmine Champa
20. Oovi	Front Mid Thigh	Letting Go	Trifolia Yarrow	Lavender Rosewood
21. Ani	Central Above Knee	Balance	Yarrow Yarrow Lavender	Rose Sandalwood
22a. Janu	Two Points Above Knee	Balance	Sandalwood Cedarwood	Yarrow Lavender
b. Janu	Two Points Below Knee	Joints	Sandalwood Cedarwood	Yarrow Lavender

MARMA POINTS (continued)

Indian Name	Location	Function/area of Body Affected	Essential Oils	
23. Unnamed	Mid Outside Shin	Kidney-Adrenal	Orange Cypress Myrtle	Cedarwood Sandalwood
24. Unnamed	Lower Inside Shin	Reproductive System	Dhavana Geranium Clary Sage	Angelica Vetiver
25. Gulpha	Inside and Outside Ankle	Reproductive System	Dhavana Clary Sage	Jatamansi Vetiver
Foot				
26. Khipram	Above and Below Where Toes Join	Sinus Lymph	Rosemary Eucalyptus	Camphor
27. Koorcha	Ball of Foot	Stomach	Keawa	Sandalwood
28. Talhridayam	Center of Foot	Heart	Rose Cardamon	Sandalwood Rosemary
29. Koorchshir	Center of Heel	Spinal Alignment 1st Chakra	Angelica Trifolia	Jatamansi Vetiver
Leg (back)				
30a. Indravastih	Center of Calf	Cramps Leg Pain	Lavender Lemongrass	Wintergreen
b. Indravastih	Lower Calf	Athletic	Lavender Lemongrass	Wintergreen
31. Janu	Behind Knee	Spleen (Left) Liver/Gall Bladder (Right)	Angelica Lemon Balm	Lemon Yarrow
32. Aanih	Lower Back of Thigh	Intestines	Trifolia Ginger	Thyme
33. Vorvee	Upper Back of Thigh	Circulation of Leg	Juniper Cypress	Eucalyptus
34. Kteektaninam	Center of Buttock	Equilibrium	Yarrow Lavender Sandalwood	Geranium Rose
Back				
35. Gudam	Tip of Tail Bone	Alignment - 1st Chakra	Vetiver Jatamansi Cypress	Labdanum Ginger

Indian Name	Location	Function/area of Body Affected	Essential Oils	
36. Kukundaraye	Top of Sacrum	Alignment - 2nd Chakra	Cypress Orange	Birch Juniper
37. Nitamba	Lower Kidney Area	Kidney	Lemongrass Juniper	Cypress Orange
38. Koopram	Upper Kidney Area	Adrenal	Angelica Lavender	Yarrow Geranium
39. Vrahti	Mid Back	Heart, Lungs	Rosemary Eucalyptus Cardamon	Camphor Rose
40. Asphalakah	Upper Back	Thymus, Heart	Thyme Yarrow	Lavender Rose
Shoulder				
41. Asaha	Top of Shoulder	Relaxes Nervous System Self Esteem	Ginger Rosewood	Sandalwood Cedarwood
42. Shaunkh	Above and in Front of Ear	Clear Hearing	Lavender Eucalyptus	Peppermint
43. Utkshepau	Above and Behind Ear	Increasing Awareness & Brain Activity	Basil Camphor	Rosemary
44. Apa	Temple	Vision	Peppermint Basil	Clary Sage Lemon
45. Sthapui	Between Eyebrows	Balancing 6th Chakra Pituitary Inner Vision	Lavender Jasmine Keawa	Camphor Basil Henna
46. Adhipati	Top of Head	Pineal Self Realization Balances 7th Chakra	Myrrh Shamama	Frankincense
47. Nadi	Back Top of Head	Posterior Pituitary	Brahmi	Sandalwood

MARMA POINTS (continued)

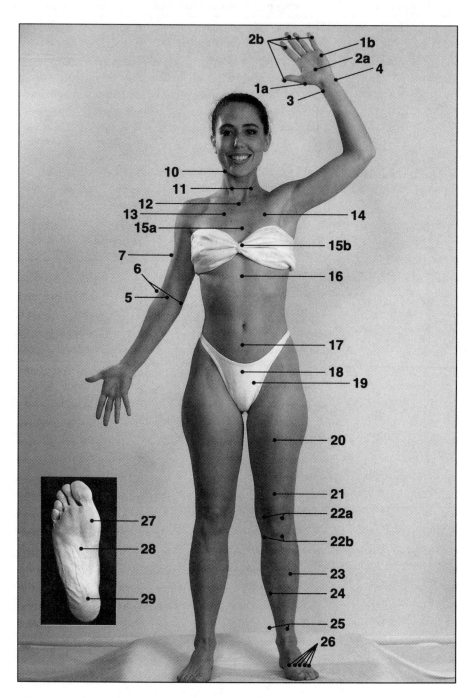

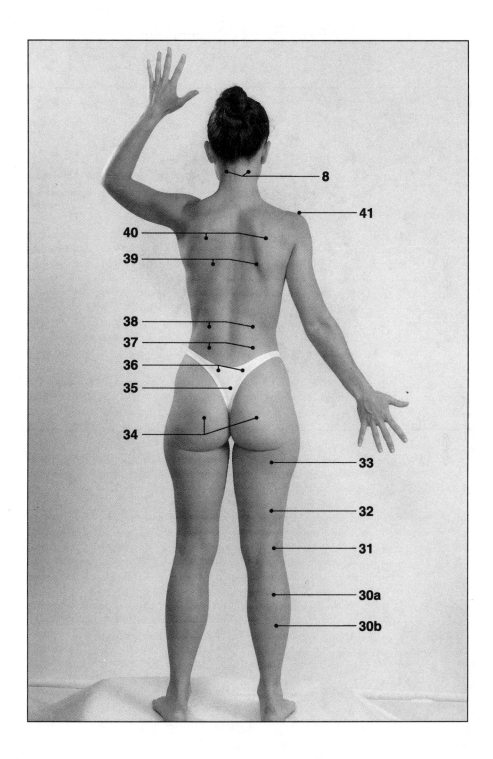

MARMA POINTS (continued)

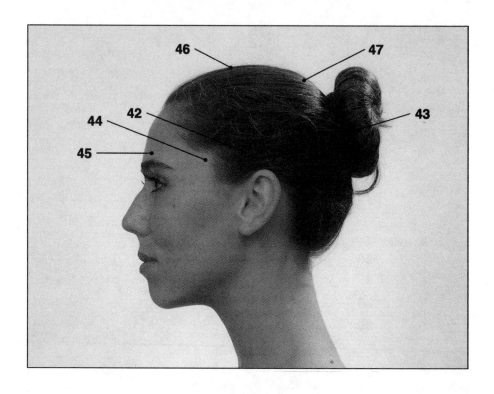

CHAPTER NINETEEN

EASY RIDER GUIDE TO TRAVEL

GENERAL PREPARATION FOR TRAVEL

The secret to traveling with a minimum of symptoms and complaints is to prepare several days in advance of your journey. It can be helpful to take 100 mg. of B complex, 3000 mg. of vitamin C, and eat foods which pacify your particular doshic imbalance. Vatas especially should eat foods which are rich and oily, Pittas should concentrate on salads and steamed vegetables, and Kaphas should scrupulously avoid oils and dairy products and eat lots of vegetables and spices. It is important for all types to drink plenty of fluids, either one-half hour before meals or three hours after meals, when your food has digested.

TRAVEL BY AIR

Essential Oils for Balancing Vata During Travel

angelica (grounding, toning, immunity)

anise (stomach problems, equilibrium)

cypress (grounding)

geranium (balancing)

ginger (balance)

grapefruit (energizing)

lavender (balancing)

rosewood (grounding)

sandalwood (grounding)

vetiver (grounding)

When traveling, Vata types typically experience constipation from disruption of their routine. External application of trifolia with vegetable oil can be of great help for all types who experience constipation. Dry skin is especially prevalent with exposure to high altitude, pressure changes, wind and sun. Eating a rich diet, full of foods with high oil content, is helpful, and frequent oiling of the skin will counter this natural tendency toward dry skin and constipation. The rush and stress of travel naturally creates anxiety for Vata types, which can result ultimately in a spaced-out, disconnected feeling. Compresses, inhalations, and washing the face with a hot, damp hand towel treated with a few drops of essential oils, can ease the anxiety and provide more centering.

How Light Travels

Bryan: Because Light frequently travels for business, she must arrive refreshed and alert. She often speaks or performs treatments the night of the day she arrives. Your typical seventeen-hour flight from Seattle to Copenhagen can leave the average traveler disoriented and non-functioning for up to three days. Before the flight, Light gives herself a complete rubdown with sesame oil mixed with liberal amounts of angelica, ginger and rosewood for grounding, to counter her Vata tendency to be spaced out and anxious. Because she is a mixed-type, experiencing Kapha congestion and fluid retention, she also adds juniper and cypress to move fluids. On the plane, every four to five hours she goes to the restroom and takes three minutes to rub down as much of her body as she is able with her mixture. She will ask the flight attendant for hot water to which she will add a drop of ginger or anise to calm her stomach. She occasionally carries a damp washcloth to which essential oils have been added and the flight attendant, if not too busy, will often heat this in the microwave for her. Because she is up all night before the flight preparing, her philosophy is to catch up on all possible sleep during the flight. She often turns down meals and just sleeps the flight away. Upon arrival at her destination, a nice long soak in an essential oil bath begins her acclimatization, and frequent use of essential oils internally and externally provide a smooth transition over the next several days.

Essential Oils for Balancing Pitta During Travel

chamomile (anti-inflammatory, calming)
cumin (digestion)
fennel (digestion, equilibrium)
geranium (relaxing)
lavender (calming, balancing)
lime (detoxification)

mint (cooling, reawakening, calming stomach)
rose (balancing, calming)
yarrow (anti-inflammatory, balancing, connecting)

When traveling, Pitta types experience irritability and anger. They take more seriously the last minute rush, have less patience with long lines, customs officials and taxi drivers. The rising fire of their irritation can make their skin more sensitive and they may experience inflammations, eruptions and a sour body odor that accompanies increased perspiration. Ultimately, their resistance to wasted time, discourtesy or inefficiency will produce fatigue. Frequent snacks before, during and after travel can help maintain blood sugar levels and moderate mood swings. Grounding oils like yarrow, geranium, rose and sandalwood can counter the Vata nature of travel, while the calming and cooling oils like mint, lavender and chamomile will keep anger and irritability to a minimum. A cool, damp washcloth imbued with essential oils can be used every few hours to relax the Pitta passenger. Luke warm or cool essential oil baths before and after travel are important, as is oiling the skin with coconut oil. Adding a drop of mint or lavender to a cold cup of water is easy, even at 20,000 feet.

Cry Baby Blues

While Light and I were traveling on a noisy, crowded flight from Tampa to Seattle, we found ourselves sitting directly in front of a very uncomfortable, unhappy, and vocal baby who cried inconsolably for the first hour of the flight. I always travel with my essential oil kit in a carry-on bag to avoid breakage from poor handling or atmospheric changes in the unpressurized baggage compartment, and I offered my most expensive rose oil to the frustrated mother as an antidote to her situation. Less than happy with my offer of assistance, and regarding my small bottle of rose oil with suspicion and contempt, she declined, even with my further assurances that it was quite natural and that I was a doctor. I don't generally believe in forcibly treating people, but after a minute of disbelief, turning into anger and resentment, and for the sake of myself, the other passengers, and the child's well being, I liberally dosed the headrest of my seat with not only rose, but also lavender and blue chamomile. The aroma was strong enough that it produced a few glances from the flight attendant and some comments from the people across the aisle, but within five minutes the baby was peacefully sleeping and the rest of the flight was uneventful. In general, you can use small amounts of essential oil in your personal aromatherapy so that it will not be offensive to nearby passengers. It is fortunate that a small amount goes a long way, and that the body and mind respond to homeopathic dilutions in the air as well as larger doses applied directly to the body.

Essential Oils for Balancing Kapha During Travel

angelica (immune stimulant)

basil (digestive, mental stimulant)

bergamot (refreshing, stimulant)

cardamon (digestant, especially in coffee)

eucalyptus (stimulant, fluid retention, decongestant)

ginger (balance, digestant, stimulant)

grapefruit (stimulant)

juniper (fluid retention, stimulant)

orange (fluid retention, stimulant)

rosemary (fluid retention, decongestant)

thyme (digestant, stimulant, immune builder)

Kapha travelers most often experience swelling and water retention, and occasionally constipation. The hustle, bustle and movement is stressful to the Kapha type who prefers to stay at home; their resistance can make them tired and lethargic. For Kapha types, vegetable oil is the least desirable carrying medium to apply essential oil onto the skin; however, mustard and canola oils are very heating vegetable oils and are suitable. Another alternative is an alcohol-based essential oil mixture or essential oil water mixture, since the water will not be absorbed by the skin and will evaporate. Strips of cloth or even cotton socks can be soaked in these mixtures and wrapped on the feet periodically for compression and increased fluid movement. Upward massage of the feet helps to move the lymph and blood, and as much walking as possible is beneficial to keep everything fluid. Warm teas with a drop of juniper, cypress or orange can keep the digestion moving. Hot essential oil baths upon arrival complete the balancing act.

Additional Flying Tips

It is important for all types, and especially Vatas, to eat root vegetables such as yams and sweet potatoes for grounding. Vatas can do an oil basti (enema) the night before. Those who experience motion sickness can use circular (Band-Aid®) patches behind the ear with lavender, ginger, anise or fennel oil. Coffee and alcohol served in airports or aboard the plane would be best avoided by all groups, although would be most tolerated by Kapha types.

OCEAN TRAVEL

Travel by boat can be distressing to anyone who experiences sea sickness. Dizziness, nausea and vomiting can occur on even the largest cruise ship. Some people feel that in Vata types seasickness is the body's reaction to fear of death, in this case by drowning. In Pitta types, seasickness can be a reaction to relinquishing all control to a greater force (mother ocean); and in Kapha types it can be a rebellion against the movement and uncertainty in a foreign environment, exacerbated by the excess mucous which Kaphas sometimes have. All types can adapt to sea travel by avoiding greasy foods, which can stay on the stomach as much as six hours, and eating frequent, small amounts of bland carbohydrates, such as crackers or bread. High doses of vitamin C before or during the journey, and the regular use of calming and balancing essential oils, especially anise, ginger, lavender and fennel, would be helpful. Many people find the "dot" patch behind the ear works, as well as Dramamine® or Scopamine® patches.

AUTOMOBILE TRAVEL

Much of the advice for other forms of transportation apply to auto travel. Preparatory vitamins, essential oil baths and skin oiling all apply. Because the car is your own micro-environment, you can be more liberal in your essential oil usage. Peppermint, basil and rosemary can counteract fatigue; a tissue or a cloth handkerchief can be dosed with essential oils and inserted into the air conditioning vent to disperse into the car. I reserve lavender for motel baths or wiping my neck and face in rest stops as it can be too relaxing for me while driving.

Motel rooms often have a musty or smoky odor left by previous travelers. In addition to spritzing the room, the air conditioners often have a plastic filter which can be removed, rinsed clean of dust and sprinkled with essential oils. Within minutes the entire room smells naturally fresh.

CHAPTER TWENTY

METAPHYSICS AND SPECIAL AYURVEDIC TREATMENTS

AURAS, CHAKRAS, AND ESSENTIAL OILS

The Bridge Between Matter and Mind, Body and Spirit

The Aura

The aura is part of our psychic anatomy, readily seen by psychics and others with special abilities. The aura radiates around us and all living things, always in constant motion, vibrating and pulsating. Our state of mind affects our aura, as do life style, emotions, thoughts, and attitudes.

The aura has three layers, or subtle bodies. The first is the etheric, composed of energy from beyond the earth. It is our celestial being. This is the force which we radiate out to others. In India it is called *prana*; the Chinese named it *chi*; and the Japanese know it as *ki*. This etheric field is about an inch from the physical body. Spritzing lotions, massage and perfume oils enhance this field. Our thoughts vibrate in this field, and the sages say that our karmic needs for certain experiences are placed here to guide us into what we came to do. Our karmic sheath comes into our mother in the seventh month and becomes part of the etheric body. This is when the soul enters the body—at this point we start working on past karma.

The second auric layer is the astral body. Astral means connected to the stars. This body helps us see the world and weave our energies through it. It extends about a foot or more out from our body and relates to our emotional states and how we behave in our daily activities. Our moods, feelings, and the energy we send to others are dictated by this body. Our illnesses are filtered down by our state of being in the astral body.

The third layer is our spirit body. It is our soul force which always is and always will be. It can project out farthest from our physical body; as much as 200 yards, depending on our spiritual development and the work we do on the earth. These three layers of the aura are connected to our physical body by the system of energetic vortices called the chakras.

Chakras

The word *chakra* comes from Sanskrit and means wheels, or vortexes. Some of the first seers were the tantric masters who developed this system. Described as wheels of force arranged vertically on the trunk and head, chakras are transfer points for our thoughts and feelings and the physical functioning of specific endocrine glands. The chakra system is the mechanism through which angry thoughts can affect liver-adrenal metabolism, for instance, or fear of speaking your truth can disturb thyroid function.

Chakras exist on the outside of the etheric body, and are points of connection through which energy flows from one being to another. This may explain why we are attracted to each other or why sometimes people just can't connect.

Chakras are like flowers on a stalk, and connect from the front of the body all the way to the back of the spine; when they are open they are like bells, and you can feel the energy. Even though you may not be able to see chakras, you might be able to feel them with your hands. When there is balance between the chakras, you have maximum vitality, health, and body ecstatic. This energy flowing is what makes it possible for our physical bodies to exist.

Chakras open and close according to our emotions; our state of mind affects whether they are glowing bright or blocked. According to a person's level of development, chakras appear in different diameters. As we work on ourselves, acquire discipline, and take time for self-development, our chakras pulsate with light. When our emotions are blocked, they become dull and sluggish.

The Seven Chakras

The first chakra resonates in men between the genitals and the anus. On a woman, the force resonates from the cervix of the uterus, which may be why women are able to give birth. The first chakra is woman's foundation, her base, her survival, how she feels about being here on the earth. When this area is blocked, women may experience constipation, hemorrhoids, low back pain, sciatica, fear, instability with money, and powerlessness, and the need to control life. When women free themselves and open this energy, they trust the universe, trust life, and are able to let go of struggle.

The second chakra represents our creative energy and is associated with the functions of our reproductive organs. It is our sexual energy. This wheel vibrates from the pubic bone and expresses out through our creative will. When blocked, we may experience lack of purpose, impotence, frigidity, cystitis, confusion, restlessness, fantasies, jealousy, guilt, and a sense that life is doing it to us. When it is open, we can experience our creativity, approaching every challenge that shows up in a creative manner. We open to, and understand, our sexuality.

The third chakra is located on the solar plexus, in the lower thoracic area and diaphragm. It is connected energetically to the functioning of the adrenals and pancreas, which regulates blood sugar. When blocked, we experience digestive problems, lust for power, and we become pushy, overbearing and egocentric. When it is open, we attune our will to the will of God. We realize nothing happens against our will; we choose peace. We embrace self discipline. We let go of beliefs that don't serve us any longer. We manifest our work easily and effortlessly. We are in full trust of the universe.

The fourth chakra is associated with the heart and thymus. It is located in the mid-chest area and reflects our connectedness. It is also the center of joining between the higher and lower chakras. When this center is closed or restricted, we experience heart problems, loneliness, isolation and hatred, and live in condemnation of others, feeling separated and disconnected. When open, we experience unconditional love. We know that love is fact and the basis of our being. We see the past and our memories as an opportunity to heal. Everyone and everything is our teacher. Our challenges are lessons and we experience connectedness to all things.

The fifth chakra is located in the throat and the neck area. When obstructed or blocked, we experience voice, hearing, and communication problems, sore throats, and difficulty expressing our feelings (telling the truth). When we open this area, we become a channel for truth. Nothing holds back our expression, "and the truth shall set us free." We speak God's truth.

The sixth chakra, or third eye, is located above or between the eyebrows, affects our receptivity and is associated with the pituitary gland. When blocked we experience vision problems, headaches, feelings of separation, fogginess, and dizziness. When open we see our connection to all things. We know the future, the past, and we live in the now. Our clairvoyance is stimulated—our ability to see and understand all things. Nothing can separate us from our source. We become a witness of the world without judgment or attachment to the outcome.

The seventh chakra is located at the crown of the head and is associated with the pineal gland. It is a source of divine energy and self realization. When it is blocked, we dwell in the ego. We pray out of desperation. We separate ourselves from God and our source. When open, the ego falls away. We become the servant of God's work here on the planet. We surrender our body to the higher power of God. We become one with all things. At this instant the energy reverses and radiates forth as light. We experience enlightenment.

Guide to the Chakras and Essential Oils

	Western Name	Sanskrit Name	Meaning	Location	Essential Oils	Color
7th	Crown	Sahasrara	Thousand petaled	Top of cranium	Violet absolute, frankincense, myrrh, shamama, hina	Violet
6th	Third Eye	Ajna	Unlimited power	Above and between eyebrows	Basil, camphor, lavender, jasmine, eucalyptus, rosemary, lemon, keawa	Indigo
5th	Throat	Vishuddha	Pure	Throat	Cajeput, sandalwood, bergamot, tea tree, blue chamomile	Blue
4th	Heart	Anahata	Unstricken	Chest over heart	Rose, cinnamon, champa, orange, neroli, bergamot, yarrow, lavender	Green
3rd	Solar Plexus	Manipura	City of gems	Between navel and ribcage	Dhavana, gold chamomile, sandalwood, anise, fennel, champa, lavender	Yellow
2nd	Sexual	Svadhishana	Dwelling place of self	Pubic area	Cedarwood, clary sage, cypress, lemon verbena, trifolia, myrtle, rosewood, ylang ylang, patchouli	Orange
1st	Base Root	Muladadhara	Foundation	Between genitals and anus	Vetiver, angelica, cypress, jatamansi, rock rose, ginger, angelica	Red

Application: Mix a total of 30% of the prescribed essential oils with 70% vegetable oil. Cold pressed vegetable oil (sweet almond, grape seed, jojoba, etc.) is preferred. Place 10 drops of this mixture on the corresponding chakra location and rub into the skin in a counter-clockwise direction while visualizing the corresponding color. Or, place a total of 6-12 drops of the prescribed essential oils into one cup of water. Soak a small cloth with the solution, squeeze out the excess and place as a warm compress over the chakra. Cover with a towel and rest until cool.

CHAKRA OILS

Essential oils increase our finest and farthest vibrations and assist all of the subtle bodies. Essential oils can stimulate and assist in the process of awakening, healing, opening the chakras, and strengthening the aura. There are many other ways chakras can be stimulated and opened—massage, acupuncture, chiropractic, breath work, visualization, and channeling energy to specific sites, to name a few. Essential oils can play a vital part in stimulating the chakra system, as essential oils are

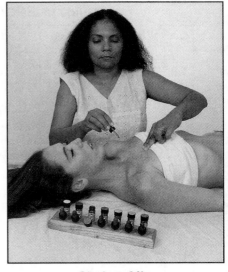

Chakra Oils

the spirit, the pranic force of a plant—and this is the plant's gift to *our* prana. You can anoint the chakras before meditation, or have another person anoint you after you have received a massage or before going to bed. Using meditation and yoga, holy men in India work for years to create these openings. We are fortunate to have all these technologies to assist us.

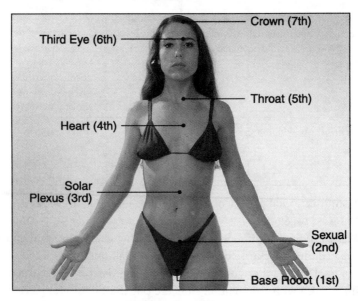

Chakra Locations

GEMSTONES AND ESSENTIAL OILS

Neil S. Cohen, in his publications *Legion of Light Guides*, tells us that crystals, gems and minerals can be tools for transformation. They are solidified reflections of those properties which are already within us. He urges us to keep this in mind as we use gems and crystals and not to give away our power. See them as an aspect of ourselves; as tools, as guides, as gifts from nature, to be enjoyed. We acknowledge the information he has collected in his *Guides* as influential in this section.

As we have said, essential oils are the etheric energy, the life force of plants. By combining the life force of plants and the mineral crystals, we can create a synergistic effect, enhancing both the energy of the stone and the energy of the oil. Once the essential oils have been potentized by the minerals—for a period of an hour, a day, a week, a month—those essential oils are transformed and now have within them the power of the stones. It is also beneficial to put a single drop of essential oil onto a gem or stone before wearing it.

The following will be a brief listing of some of the more common gemstones and essential oils that can be used by the various dosha types to create a synergistic effect. The information that follows is intuitive and esoteric knowledge and is not hard science nor a replacement for herbal, aromatherapy or medical treatment. Although specific oils are named, any oil can be energized by any stone.

Agate is especially good for Vata because of its grounding qualities, yet it still allows excitement and energetics to continue.

Vata: bergamot. Pitta: champa and keawa. Not recommended for Kapha.

Amber is a fossil resin that offers protection from negative energies, assists with anxiety, nervousness, tension and cramping. It is very calming to the nervous system, assists with meditation, helps open to guidance, enhances the ability to channel and use other psychic abilities. It is wonderful for children in their development.

Vata: rosewood, angelica, musk and chamomile. Pitta: shamama, sandalwood, lavender, basil, calamus, gotu kola (brahmi) and mint. Not best for Kapha.

Amethyst improves immune function and enhances the endocrine glands, especially the pineal and pituitary. It calms the nervous system, assists in transformation, protects the aura and enhances intuitive qualities.

Vata: rosewood, brahmi, basil. Pitta: neroli and rose. Kapha: calamus.

Aquamarine is highly astringent and reduces fluid retention. It is relaxing to the nervous system and sends energy to the urinary tract, easing fears. Balancing to the liver, it also banishes anger. Excellent for the verbal expression of will.

Vata: rosemary, eucalyptus, gold chamomile and basil. Pitta: blue chamomile, cajeput, birch, wintergreen. Kapha: rosemary, juniper and cypress.

Azurite is a relaxant to the nervous system. Helps to purify the blood. Enhances your intuition and psychic abilities.

Vata: basil and angelica. Pitta: lavender and blue chamomile. Kapha: niaouli, fir, and lemon.

Benitoite is excellent for senility, thyroid problems and aids in the assimilation of calcium. Helps regulate weight.

Vata: galbanum, vanilla, mace, angelica. Pitta: lilac, violet and tuberose. Kapha: orange.

Betyl is excellent for constipation and digestion, releases fear, assists with moving forward and letting go of the past.

Vata: trifolia, lemon and ginger. Pitta: peppermint, immortelle. Kapha: cubeb, black pepper and ginger.

Blue Sapphire helps to reduce fever and infection, soothes anger, helps with weight loss, arthritis, auto-immune disease, paralysis, inflammation, thyroid conditions and excess bleeding.

Vata: gold chamomile, valerian, cypress. Pitta: blue chamomile, Moroccan chamomile and geranium. Kapha: seaweed absolute, garlic, onion, myrtle.

Carnelian brings energy to the urinary tract, respiratory tract and digestive tract. Assists healing, gives energy to the aura. Assists in the assimilation of vitamins and minerals.

Vata: dhavana, angelica, allspice, orange, bergamot. Pitta: rose, lemongrass. Kapha: myrrh, orange, juniper and cypress.

Cat's Eye is a warming stone which increases the mental forces and helps open psychic abilities. It supports spiritual energies and is a relaxant to the nervous system.

Vata: hina and dhavana. Not recommended for Pitta. Kapha: trifolia, lotus seed and basil.

Celestite is a stress reducer, and brings peace of mind. It enhances the thyroid and is best used over the neck area. Celestite opens the throat chakra and enhances clear communications and truth.

Vata: bergamot. Pitta: tea tree, sandalwood, blue chamomile. Kapha: cajeput

Citrine, with its yellow color, is associated with balancing the forces of will and helping to open to the abundance of life and to the lighter side of life's experiences. It is one of the best stones for lowering Vata. It can be a muscle stimulant, a nerve relaxant, and is good for back pain and headaches, and strengthening to the digestive system and the urinary tract.

Vata: eucalyptus, anise. Citrine can be irritating to Pitta, but may be occasionally used with keawa, fennel and myrtle. Kapha: rosemary, calamus and mugwort.

Coral helps with mineral imbalances, inflammation, and swelling, and is a balancer to the blood. It brings stability, sexual enhancement, opens the heart, and assists in manifestation.

Vata: jatamansi, rosewood, dhavana. Pitta: clary sage, chamomile. Kapha: juniperberry, eucalyptus, and rosemary.

Diamond is known to amplify whatever energy you are currently running in your body. It enhances perception, the reproductive system, the immune system, and can be excellent for diseases such as AIDS, cancer, and diabetes. A well-made zirconium can be a substitute.

Vata: angelica, cardamon, frankincense and sandalwood. Pitta: brahmi oil, immortelle, yarrow. Kapha: chamomile, elecampane and myrrh.

Garnet is a balancing stone for all doshas. It is excellent for depression and helps restrain the ego. It assists in letting go of illusionary reality.

Vata: amber blend. Pitta: rose, lavender and sandalwood. Kapha: lemon and basil.

Jade was thought by the Orientals to increase fertility. Its green color helps to reduce fever and excess heat. It creates alignment between the heart and the emotions.

It is not the best stone for Vata. Pitta: it can be enhanced with lavender, rose, sandalwood, yarrow and geranium. Kapha: orange, eucalyptus, juniper and cypress.

Lapis Lazuli stimulates the lymphatic system, helps to build the endocrine system, and works especially with the pituitary. It is energizing to the expression of thoughts and all levels of communication.

Vata: rosewood, bay, brahmi, angelica, frankincense. Pitta: peppermint, rose and sandalwood. Kapha: cumin, camphor and orange.

Moonstone has many similar properties to pearl and the same oils can be applied to its use.

Opal is stimulating to the pituitary. It is an immune balancer, helps to open the heart chakra and contact the higher self.

Vata: rosewood and cardamon. Pitta: sandalwood, yarrow, lavender, rose geranium. Kapha: jatamansi, sandalwood, and orange.

Pearl is a mineral gift from the water environment. It helps to regulate the fluid movement in the muscle tissues of the body, and relaxes the mind into being secure with its knowing.

Vata: ginger, lavender, lemongrass, parsley and valerian. Pitta: chamomile, lemon balm, lemongrass, lavender and yarrow. Kapha: anise, basil, elecampane and parsley.

Quartz enhances the immune system and hormone system. It regulates, balances and tones the body. It increases all communications, and magnifies anything which is already occurring.

Works with all oils.

Rose Quartz is helpful with urinary tract infections. Assists in relieving fear, anger, resentment, guilt. It is cooling and calming.

Excellent for Pitta: blue chamomile, rose, mint, lavender and sandalwood. Not recommended for Vata and Kapha.

Ruby is a regulator of the heart. It improves digestion, assists with developing your will forces, provides vitality, and security in survival issues.

Vata: rose and lavender. Not the best stone for Pitta. Kapha: orange and cypress.

Turquoise aids in circulation, helps with the lungs and heart, brings energy to the nervous system and enhances communication.

Vata: cardamon, cinnamon, bergamot. Pitta: lavender, geranium. Kapha: orange and cypress.

ESSENTIAL OILS AND PANCHA KARMA

Seasonal Housecleaning

It seems incredible that ancient peoples developed awareness of the body's systems and created techniques for cleansing each one. Records indicate that pancha karma was in practice as early as 300 AD. Many variations of pancha karma have developed but all forms seek to purify and open the blocked channels of the body as a basis for health and rejuvenation. Traditionally, pancha karma was performed at the turn of the seasons to prepare the body for changes in diet and environment. In other words, the body is the temple of the soul. Keep it clean.

Pancha karma is carefully adapted for each body type and for specific conditions. The five actions to purify the body are **Oelation** (*snehana*), **Purgation** (*virechana*), **Sweats** (*svedhana*), **Enema** (*basti*) and **Nasal Therapy** (*nasya*). Some systems include **Emesis** (vomiting), **Bloodletting**, **Shirodhara**, and **Tarpana** (relationship healing).

In chronic disease, the blockages of the channels brought on by narrow, selfish and self-indulgent lifestyles, produce symptoms of pain and dysfunction—a cry for change. As the channels open, the individual opens to connection (love) of self, of others and for all existence. As you purify, you open to the Healer within. As you connect and realize that separation is an illusion, service to others is a natural end result. Nature can give you a second chance in life (rejuvenation - longevity) as an opportunity to give back to life what you have received.

Oelation (snehana)

Oelation involves both the external application of oils to the body, and taking oils internally to soften and make supple the tissues of the body, so that ama (toxins) can flow freely outward.

Internal Application: two to four tablespoons of castor oil, ghee or medicated oils are consumed for several days to prepare the digestive tract for cleansing. Due to the lack of medicated oils available in this country, and the time it takes to prepare them at home, essential oils added to vegetable oil give you a substitute less likely to be rancid from long storage or shipping, yet full of active healing properties.

Vata responds best to castor oil, sesame oil, or ghee, with one drop of (choose one) ginger, jatamansi, dhavana, sandalwood, angelica or trifolia.

Pitta oils include ghee or olive oil with one drop of (choose one) mint, lavender, coriander, chamomile, turmeric, sandalwood. Fresh aloe or aloe-olive medicated oil is also excellent.

Kaphas do well with castor, mustard, canola or almond oils with one drop added of juniper, basil, turmeric, ginger, orange or lemon.

External Application: loosens and softens the external channels —pores, sebaceous glands, lymph and capillaries—and prepares them for cleansing through sweating. The same base oils mentioned above are used with higher concentrations of the same essential oils (30 - 100 drops per 4 oz. bottle). The oil is applied liberally, worked into the surface of the skin, allowed to absorb. Kapha types do best with less base oil and higher concentrations of essential oils.

Purgation (virechana)

Purgation is accomplished with laxative herbs which cleanse the small intestine and reduce excess fire. Mild purgatives such as castor oil with aloe are appropriate in Vata types. Stronger purgatives are more appropriate for Pitta, such as aloe, gentian, rhubarb; and for Kapha, senna, rhubarb, aloe. Purgation is practiced for two days, as more would lower the digestive fire and deplete the vital forces. Essential oils play no part in internal purgation; however, to stimulate elimination you can perform abdominal massage, in a clockwise direction, using two tablespoons vegetable oil and 30 drops (total) of any of the following essential oils, alone or in combination: rosemary, lemon, peppermint, patchouli, cedarwood, angelica, lavender, thyme, geranium, mandarin, tangerine, Roman chamomile, fennel, or ginger.

Sweats (svedhana)

After the skin is oiled, the skin channels are open, supple, and ready to eliminate wastes. Sweats use the natural forces of heat and steam to open the outer channels and aid the body's natural eliminative processes; ¼ of all waste exits through the skin. Essential oils added to the steam bring life force to the process, stimulating and energizing the skin. A steam cabinet, where your head remains outside and cool, is the best type of steam. The genitals and heart area can be protected from the heat with small, cool, damp towels. Some sources recommend dry heat during early elimination, switching to moist sauna when the channels have been cleared.

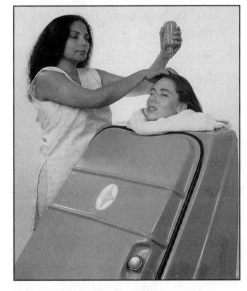

It is important that Vata types not do sweats excessively, and drink a lot of water to replace the fluids lost. Pitta types should do sweats at lower temperature and for less time than other doshas. Kapha types need svedhana

Steam Cabinet

the most and can benefit by higher temperatures and longer times.

Oils for the Sauna: mix 10-20 drops (total) with water for steaming:

Vata: cardamon, ginger, eucalyptus, cinnamon, chamomile, jatamansi, valerian

Pitta: yarrow, coriander, lavender, chamomile, cumin, anise, fennel, lime, mint

Kapha: cypress, juniper, black pepper, eucalyptus, rosemary, orange, yarrow, bay

After sauna it is important to wrap up in a sheet or blanket, lie down, and allow the body temperature to slowly lower to normal. Heat raises the metabolic rate, increasing elimination of wastes and stimulating immune response.

The excess oil on the body contains wastes and should be removed by showering and scrubbing with mild PH-balanced soap or shampoo, vigorous toweling, or powdering the body with chana (chick pea flour); allow it to absorb the oils then remove it.

Heat and the Immune System

There was a swampy region of Italy where, early in this century, most of the inhabitants suffered malarial fevers, but cancer was almost unknown. When the swamps were drained, malaria disappeared but the cancer rate rose to nationwide levels. Science began to explore the role of fevers and heat in immune response. A new medical experimental therapy involves removing the blood, one pint at a time, heating it, which destroys viruses and bacteria, cooling it, and returning it to the body. Why not do saunas?

Enema (basti)

Traditional Western enemas, using plain water, are drying and deplete the colon. Ayurveda uses herbal teas, medicated oils and vegetable oils, milk and yogurt to cleanse, build and nourish the sensitive and important eliminative tract.

Vata dryness often extends into the large intestine. Oils such as flax and sesame, plain yogurt, and nourishing-demulcent teas such as mullein, licorice, comfrey root, flax seed, slippery elm and aloe (fresh gel), and heating herbs such as cardamon, cinnamon, and ginger, are used instead of water. To these can be added 10 drops per gallon of any Vata-reducing essential oils.

Pitta heat requires cooling herb tea and milk to which can be added ten drops of Pitta-reducing essential oils per gallon.

Kapha colons usually have excess mucous buildup, so oil, milk or other dairy products are not advised. Teas can be made with a combination of one or more of the following herbs: aloe, rosemary, bala, manjista, haritaki, anise, amalaki, eucalyptus, juniper, ginger, prickly ash, fennel, ajwan, cinnamon. Coffee can be an especially good additive with up to ten drops (total) of the following essential oils: ajwan, anise, bay, cardamon, elecampane, eucalyptus, ginger, lemongrass, myrrh, orange, sage.

Administration

In ancient times basti was administered using a long, hollowed-out, trailing gourd or a clay pot to which a hollow reed was attached. Today an enema bag will suffice, although I prefer the colema board system because it allows the patient to receive and release up to five gallons of basti mixture while relaxing over the toilet. When visiting the Ghandi Center in India, Light saw basti equipment very similar to the Colema Board. The Colema Board was developed by Dr. Bernard Jensen, D.C., a world traveler. While searching for healing secrets, he probably saw similar devices.

With a traditional enema, 1-2 quarts may be received and held for up to 30 minutes, utilizing shoulder stands or slant board positions to assist retention, after which the patient must get up, walk to the toilet and release the mixture. During administration, the stomach should be massaged counterclockwise to move the mixture through the colon; then massage the abdomen in a clockwise direction to assist release. The mixture should be warm but not hot. If the patient experiences pressure or discomfort, the flow should be stopped until massage and breathing releases the spasms.

Nasal Therapy (nasya)

Nasya is used to clear impurities from the head and sinus, reduce pain, and promote relaxation. The stimulation of the limbic system (primitive brain) via the olfactory nerve can have profound effects on our mood, emotions, desires, appetites and memories. Powders, oils, teas or smoke are various mediums for directly affecting the prana Vata. Application of medicated oils to the ears is often included in nasal therapy. Melanie Sachs' book *Ayurvedic Beauty Care* gives a wonderful recipe for a ginger tea nasya. The *Yoga of Herbs* gives a list of herbs for smoking or inhaling.

Medicated oils are the most traditional form of nasya; the problem of availability can be circumvented by using essential oils. The basic recipe for the essential oil mixture is 1 to 3 drops of essential oil to ¼ oz. vegetable oil. Appropriate vegetable oils and essential oils are based on Dosha imbalance.

Vata: calamus, jatamansi, vetiver

Pitta: mint, coriander, rose, lavender, yarrow

Kapha: rosemary, basil, orange, eucalyptus

All: sandalwood

Administration of Nasya

The following is a Western adaptation of ancient techniques and is best performed at the end of a full-body massage that is given with medicated or essential blended massage oil. A good neck and face massage would be an acceptable alternative. Have your chosen vegetable-essential oil mixture, an eye dropper, and several small cloths or towels ready. The patient's neck should be supported, using a rolled-up towel 4-5" in diameter. The oil should be

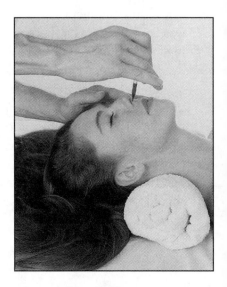

Nasal Therapy

warm, but not hot: approximately 102° F. It is appropriate to first test on oneself anything you may be giving to others.

Administration: Gently close one nostril and place 5 drops of the oil mix into the other nostril as the patient inhales. Instruct the patient to take three forceful inhalations to send the oil deep into the nasal passageway. Massage the forehead, gently around the eye socket, on and around the nose and under and on the cheek bone. Treat the opposite nostril in the same way. The patient may experience a mild burning, warmth, a sensation of inner light, of awareness, opening or release of emotions, or a sense of peace. It is reported that periodic nasya will eliminate eye puffiness and dark circles, and improve smell and taste.

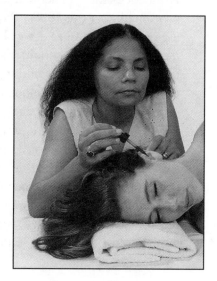

Ear Oiling

To oil the ears, turn the patient on his or her side and apply 10-15 drops of warm oil into the ear canal. Massage around auricle, and, grasping the lobe, stretch the ear gently in clockwise and counter-clockwise movements. Allow to remain 2-20 minutes then turn head to opposite side (and drain into cloth). Do opposite ear. This treatment may be useful for ear itching, pain, ringing or hearing loss.

Other Related Therapies

Emesis

Therapeutic vomiting is especially useful in Kapha imbalance and will result in excess mucous, which has collected in the stomach (usually from lung and sinus drainage), being ejected from the body. This will allow more efficient digestion and absorption of nutrients. Not to be practiced by the lay practitioner, emesis must be done under the supervision of a trained Ayurvedic practitioner as there are many contraindications. Excess vomiting can be damaging to the upper gastro-intestinal tract and nervous system. Vomiting is the body's natural reaction to sickness or poisoning and emesis is an encouragement of that reaction. Warm salt water and a finger in the throat can be used in emergency situations, but I will refrain from any further recommendations here.

Blood-Letting (*rakta moksha*)

A practice since ancient times, the letting of blood as a remedy to illness continued into the 1800s. Physicians were once called *leeches* due to their use of this creature to draw blood. Incredibly, leeches are still used by some medical doctors for conditions of hemorrhage and fluid retention just under the skin. Medicine has nothing else that works as well. Three results can be encouraged by modern bloodletting (donation of blood): someone else's life may be saved by your donation, toxins which your body has not eliminated will be directly removed, and your circulatory and immune system will be stimulated to produce fresh, new blood by the slight but sudden loss of fluid.

Essential oils can be an indirect help during blood donation. Several drops of lavender and cajeput can be used on the bandage to cover the wound, disinfect, and promote healing. One drop angelica can be taken in tea (or on the tongue) to strengthen your resolve beforehand. Anise or fennel used similarly can settle a nervous stomach. Chamomile, lemon and thyme are recommended to rebuild the blood.

Shirodhara

Shirodhara is the administering of a stream of warm oil onto the third eye area of the forehead. Traditionally, sesame oil is used, but oils appropriate to the doshic imbalance and blended with appropriate essential oils will be more effective. Shirodhara is deeply stimulating to the nervous system, re-leasing neuro-hormones and creating ecstatic feelings of relaxation and pleasure.

In India, elaborate equipment (brass pots which hang from the ceiling) is used, which can be approximated here by purchasing a separation funnel and stand from a chemistry supply. This allows a quart of oil to be *streamed* onto the forehead for half an hour. One patient described shirodhara as "dental flossing of the brain," others have described sixth Chakra orgasms; but all agree that afterwards they are left with a deep sense of connectedness, centeredness, and calm knowing. The full effect requires thirty minutes of shirodhara, but five to ten minutes administered with a one to two cup, squirt-top, plastic, massage-oil bottle is an exquisite experience. I anticipate that experiencing an abbreviated shirodhara will encourage people to pursue the complete treatment.

Application: Best administered after a massage or tarpana ceremony, when the patient is relaxed and calm. The patient is positioned on his or her back with the head at the end of the massage table. The neck is supported by a rolled-up towel, and the head is tilted back and extended off the table. The patient should be covered with a sheet or blanket, and a bolster placed under the knees. A large bowl is placed on the floor to catch the oil as it streams off the forehead. Test the temperature of the oil on the inside of your forearm.

Begin with a small stream in the center of the forehead. It is pleasurable to slowly move the stream left and right so that the entire forehead and top of head is stimulated, but most focus should be on the third eye, one inch above and between the eyebrows. Be careful that oil does not flow or spatter into the eyes. Some practitioners cover the eyes with cotton patches or cloth. When concluded, remove excess oil from forehead and hair with a small towel. Allow the patient to remain resting 5-30 minutes in a state of deep relaxation. The patient will have been advised to plan for only light activity for several hours afterwards.

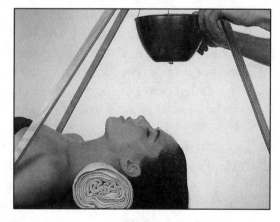

Shirodhara

Tarpana

While it is true that food, herbs, oils and lifestyles are important healing modalities to be embraced, we should acknowledge that our thoughts and feelings regarding our level of connectedness, may be the most powerful factor in our well-being.

We in the West often consider the Eastern belief of ancestor worship to be very primitive. It has long been a practice in the Catholic church on All Souls Day for families to go to the cemeteries, sit by the graves of ancestors, bring them plates of food, and have conversations with them. This is also a practice within the Hawaiian community and certain tribes of Native Americans.

However, here in the West, science has taught us that through genetic transfer from our ancestor, we have very detailed and voluminous coded information contained within our chromosomes. Eye color, height, emotional patterns, even ways of perceiving the world, may all have been given to us genetically. Some of those gifts we may enjoy, such as our grandfather's artistic ability, while others may be more of a challenge, like our mother's violent temper.

The Ceremony

The ceremony is best conducted when you are alone and relaxed. It may be helpful to dim the lights—light a candle, and perhaps burn some incense. A favorite essential oil or an oil that brings up memories from the past may be used in an aromatherapy lamp or diffuser. It is very useful to employ a method of breathing called "the re-birthing breath," or alternatively, the connected breath. This is done by breathing in through the nose and breathing out through the mouth, allowing the inhalation to be connected to the exhalation, and placing no control at all on the exhalation portion of the breath; just allowing it to lead you at its own pace, like a sigh at the end of a long day.

Starting with your mother or father, call forth each ancestor in turn. With each one, visualize them standing directly in front of you, looking into your eyes. If you did not know them personally, recall what they looked like from pictures, or remember what you heard about them. Visualize them to be in an open and receptive state, ready to hear anything that you have to say.

In the first stage of clearing, say to them: "What I want you to know is [*thought or feeling*]." Use this as an opportunity to tell them what you have felt about them, or about any of the gifts or the genetic tendencies you inherited from them. Explore with them whether or not you consider yourself to be a victim. Examine aloud what your payoff may have been in this.

Did we use this as an opportunity to indulge in self pity, or blame our problems on others? Take this as an opportunity to forgive yourself for your part in the co-creation.

Look and see if you're willing to forgive your ancestor for anything they might have done—forgiveness from the place of leaving it behind in your energetics and not carrying it with you anymore. Look into yourself, and see if you can turn what was once adversity into a catalyst for growth.

From this new place, this new point of view, reach within yourself for a willingness to thank them for the gift that they have given to you—the co-created experiences, however these may have originally appeared to you. Say, "I have learned from this experience, I have grown, I thank you."

And finally, as a symbol of a new healing that is between you and your ancestor, in your mind's eye offer them a serving of their favorite food or drink, or something they would have enjoyed eating. See them taking this from your hand, consuming it and smiling. Then look directly into their eyes and listen with your mind, and see if you can hear them giving you a blessing. Hear them wishing you success in life; wishing you to find your path, freeing you from any obligation you may have thought you had to them, freeing you to pursue your passion and your purpose. Accept this blessing and visualize them walking off into the light of their own path. Bless their path as they leave.

Bring forward each of your other ancestors, in turn, as far back as you can remember. You can do this with anyone you've been in a relationship with: brothers, sisters, friends and old lovers. This is a way to free yourself from the constraining, disbelieving thoughts that you have embraced about your relationship with others. It is an opportunity to see that you are always connected with everyone at all times, and that it is possible to change how you view the world—and how you feel about yourself and your connection to it. This is the time when you can claim your power as a co-creator.

End your tarpana session by being very still and saying the deepest and strongest affirmations that you now know to be true about yourself: I am love, I am one with all things, I am peace, I am joy, I am prosperity, I am forgiveness, I am trust, I am fulfillment, etc. And so it is.

RASAYANA

Rasayana is the Ayurvedic science of rejuvenation, longevity and immortality. For those that wish to pursue it, the goal of eternal life is considered attainable.

Much more than physical health, Ayurveda begins with healing inherited genetic physical weakness. Knowing your weaknesses by studying the diseases which your forebears have suffered, allows you to practice the lifestyle regimens which guard those faults—cracks—in your being, and use herbs and essential oils to heal and mend those weaknesses. If you know that your mother and grandmother had tendencies toward constipation, then you can adapt your eating and drinking habits and use the appropriate herbs and oils (i.e., trifolia-aloe) for healing.

Secondly, Ayurvedic balancing of the doshas ensures that excess doshic forces will not wear away at your life forces. Ayurvedic author Robert Svoboda says that if you have no weaknesses (faults), even the doshas can increase or decrease in any proportion without affecting your health. Also, if you have severe weaknesses, you will suffer no disease if you can guard your doshic balance. But most humans have inherited weakness and do *not* guard this balance, so they suffer disease.

Pancha karma is the seasonal housecleaning which allow our sins of excess indulgence and imbalance to be cleared from our beings. A physical forgiveness, we return our body to a pure state and are given a new chance at health. Tarpana is the ceremonial housecleaning of our thoughts about our ancestors and a deep healing of our genetic tendencies. Using forgiveness, tarpana becomes a most powerful tool for transformation; we let go of thoughts and feelings of fear and lack and allow ourselves to embrace love and connectedness. Modern adaptations of tarpana have extended it to include healing all our relationships, dispelling any illusion of separateness.

Rasayana is the culmination of Ayurvedic wisdom. The herbs and oils used for rejuvenation and longevity are combined with clearing of the channels, body work, meditative practices, mantra exercises and breathing (all the Vedic sciences) to create an eternal being.

Rasayana oils have properties beyond physical healing. They heal deep emotions, improve the harmony of the mind, and contain a spiritual energy which help propel you from the attachments of physical existence and separation into the deep identification with eternal principles and oneness.

Rasayana oils have special properties that allow us to transform our body-mind, to switch our cognitive operation from our primitive brain based on desire and fear, to the highest possible levels of human consciousness.

While we list rasayana oils for specific dosha types, remember that in balance, any type can use any rasayana oil.

Rasayana Oils

Vata: ajwan, aloe vera, angelica, calamus, carrotseed, Himalayan cedarwood, elecampane, frankincense, geranium, ginger, gotu kola (brahmi), jasmine, jatamansi, lotus, myrrh, rose, saffron, sandalwood, spikenard, vetiver.

Pitta: aloe vera, Himalayan cedarwood, gotu kola, jasmine, lotus, saffron.

Kapha: aloe vera, angelica, calamus, Himalayan cedarwood, elecampane, frankincense, jasmine, lotus, myrrh, rose, saffron, spikenard.

KAYA KALPA
The Bodies' Transformation

Ten thousand years ago, a king of India had a problematic, headstrong daughter, who refused to marry any of the eligible princes who were presented to her. In anger and frustration, the king decreed that she was to be blindfolded and placed in the castle courtyard in the midst of all her suitors. The man she touched was to be her husband and their children would continue the royal line.

On that day an elderly holy man wandered into the courtyard to deliver herbs to the King's physician and, by chance, was touched first by the princess. Even though he pled exemption due to his advanced age and holy vows, the King's word was law and they were to marry in three months time. The holy man consulted his teacher about his problem, and the teacher instituted an intensive program to rejuvenate and energize.

For 90 days the holy man ate a special diet, performed breathing techniques, took ritual herbal baths and was anointed with sacred oils. At the end of that time his hair had turned from gray to black, a new set of teeth had grown into his mouth, and his skin and body were youthful and strong. He married the Princess. They had many children and lived happily ever after.

This was the beginning of *kaya kalpa* (bodies' transformation), a secret healing technique used in India for thousands of years by religious healers to rejuvenate and give longevity to royalty and holy sages. Vigorously suppressed by the British, this knowledge was almost lost. There are now only 18 practitioners left in the world; fortunately, in a form more appropriate to Western life styles. In addition to its rejuvenating qualities, kaya kalpa is useful in expanding awareness, consciousness, and can be an aid in making decisions and life changes.

The Treatment

1. Begin with an assessment of the person's Ayurvedic type using pulse diagnosis and a questionnaire to discover which of the ten metabolic types the patient most closely resembles. This determines the lifestyle, diet, herbs and essential oils to bring the patient back into balance.

2. An herbal paste made from 108 Indian herbs is then applied to the entire body while the patient maintains a tantric, connective breath. The paste is specifically formulated for metabolic type, and draws out impurities while re-vitalizing the skin. The removal process reveals sites of inflammation, and concentrates stimulation to these areas while removing old skin. Skin brushing completes the stimulation and cleansing. A special herbal oil is formulated and applied to nourish the skin and a stream of hot oil is directed onto the area of the third eye, creating ecstatic sensations and expanded awareness.

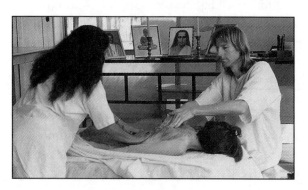

Herbal Paste

3. A hot bath using herbal extracts and aroma therapeutics, accompanied by Breath of Fire (*kundalini*) and primal sounds, creates a fiery state to release unexpressed emotions and fears, establishing a balanced receptiveness. Forgiveness rituals release the patient from past projections and create an opening for new ways of perceiving all relationships. A cooling shower returns the person to the body and initiates divine connectedness.

4. The patient is then placed in a cocoon of sheets and blankets, the chakras are anointed with the most powerful and spiritual of essential oils, and a deep meditative breath is maintained. After the treatment, the patient rests from two to five hours. A restful state of bliss is obtained that carries over in the next few days and weeks and even months in everything planned and performed.

Originally and traditionally, this treatment was conducted periodically during three months of isolation in which the patient ate a special diet, performed prescribed meditations, and lived alone in a special hut.

Today, transformation is produced by receiving a series of up to ten treatments. The purpose is to take the patient to a place within that he or she can return to at any time through the use of breath, essential oils, baths and meditation.

This treatment is for those who are prepared for transformation, and is best for those who have a spiritual practice or spiritual understanding.

The Incredible Life of Tapaswiji Majaraj
1770-1955

Born a prince in a Sikh kingdom in northern India, Tapaswiji Majaraj was trained to be a military leader, and assumed the role upon his fathers passing. At the age of 55, he tragically lost all his immediate family, and in his devastation renounced all worldly possessions. He found a guru, learned many yoga practices, and began to live a severe, austere life. He lived in a cave without food for six years, subjecting his body to extremes of heat and cold, and holding uncomfortable postures for long periods of time. During one twenty-four-year period, he remained standing or walking with his left hand over his head. He spent periods of three, seven, and eight years standing in a single spot. For twelve years he spent six hours a night meditating by a freezing lake wearing only a loin cloth while his disciples poured buckets of frigid water over his head. Those twelve summers he spent six hours each day in the scorching sun, surrounded by a ring of fire.

By the time he reached 100, his body was ruined; partially deaf and blind, no teeth, bent over at the waist, using a cane to walk, he prepared to die. On his final journey, he met a Yogi who, sensing his spiritual greatness, convinced him to undergo 90 days of kaya kalpa. He emerged looking like a man of thirty, with black hair, new teeth, and a supple strong body. After returning the favor to the Yogi (90 days of kaya kalpa service), he set out on even more austere practices. Twice more during his long life, he underwent kaya kalpa to rejuvenate his battered body, allowing him to travel, teach and demonstrate spiritual attainment and detachment to thousands.

At age 185 he demonstrated his final control over his weak, diseased and wasted body; he momentarily transformed himself into an erect, strong and radiant being, chanted the sacred AUM, and died instantly.

SUMMARY

We anticipate that the reader has found Ayurveda to be a common-sense, lay person's system for self healing. Aromatherapy, the use of essential oils, brings the most powerful concentration of healing plants right to our fingertips for instant use. The oils are easy to carry, with an indefinite shelf life, and, coupled with the information in this book, a small collection of essential oils can become a full pharmacy in any household

Ayurveda and aromatherapy can lower healthcare costs and provide effective treatment with fewer side effects, and greater patient awareness and responsibility.

Essential oils and Ayurveda have added richness and deep understanding to every aspect of our lives. In a world that needs healing in so many ways, we hope that our contribution to the joining of these sciences will help bring about individual and planetary evolution.

SECTION IV

MONOGRAPHS

INTRODUCTION

USING THE MONOGRAPHS

The monographs in this section contain information about essential oils and the plants of origin, plant families, botanical name and common name, and may be used as a quick reference to each oil's effect on the doshas, its taste, its effect on the body, the oil's energy, its action, the bodily tissues most affected, symptoms leading to use of the oil, warnings, if any, and possible applications. The information will be presented in the following order:

Common Name The name under which the oil will most often be found.

Family Name Plant families often share therapeutic properties. Knowing that a specific essential oil is part of a family can tell you a lot about how to use the oil. See Oil Families and Commonalities, page 219.

Botanical Name Specifically identifies genus and species, in case of confusion in common names.

Other Name Occasionally oils may be listed under location of origin or distillation process.

Dosha Effect   The effect the oil will have in balancing the doshas. Abbreviations are as follows:

V=Vata; P=Pitta; K=Kapha.

    – : use of the oil will tend to lower the designated dosha

    + : to use the oil will increase the dosha forces in the body

    o : no change

    + (in excess): the oil will cause dosha increase if used in excess

    VPK = means balancing to all doshas

Taste   The tastes contained in an oil will help the reader determine its dosha effect (see Chapter Three); i.e., pungent (hot) taste causes VK to diminish and P to increase because VK are cold and P is hot.

Post Digestive (PD)
Taste/Effect   This is the cumulative effect the oil will have on the body after digestion and assimilation. For instance, sweet will add tissue to the body and pungent takes away substance by increasing metabolism.

Energy   Every oil will heat or cool, help hold moisture, or create dryness.

Actions   These are the therapeutic properties of the oil (see table of essential oil therapeutics, Chapter Eleven.

Tissues   The tissues most impacted by the oil.

Indications   Symptoms for which each oil may be of benefit.

Warnings   Specific uses or circumstances requiring caution, or to be avoided.

Usage   How the oil is best applied.

Description of Aroma   With thanks and acknowledgment, all essential oil aroma descriptions are credited to Steffan Arctander, *Perfume and Flavor Material of Natural Origin.* Unless noted otherwise, no one else in the field had the range of experience to systematically describe the aromas of the oils.

Mixes Well With   Suggests other oils that work therapeutically with, or blend well with, the oil described.

OIL FAMILIES AND COMMONALITIES

It can be helpful to know that an oil is part of a plant family. Just as understanding our own family helps us to understand our nature, plant families share many therapeutic properties, and by knowing them, you better understand the individual oil. For instance, if you know that ajwan is in the carrot family, you can be sure it will be carminative, stimulating and an immune builder, just like the twelve other umbelliferaes. Listed below are ten families which happen to include sixty major plants used in making essential oils.

Burseraceae (Resin Family) - Made from the resin exudates (drippings) of desert trees and shrubs. *Frankincense, myrrh, elemi*—all the oils from this family are excellent for meditation. Coming from the tropical desert, they bring heat, contain energy to move fluids, cleanse infection, heal wounds, and build strength in the blood.

Compositae (Sunflower Family) - *Chamomile, immortelle, tansy, tarragon, dhavana, yarrow, tagetes, elecampane*—most of these oils are made from soothing flowers and are known to be healers of the skin, nerves, blood and bones. Sedating to the nerves and emotions, they are known anti-inflammatories, immune builders, and cleansers.

Coniferae-Pinaceae (Pine Family) - *Fir, cedar, cypress, juniper, pine, amber*—these oils are made from the strong aromatic wood, sap or fresh needles. They are all strong, hot, antiseptic, fluid-moving, possible skin irritants, clarifying, and grounding to the mind.

Graminae (Grass Family) - *Citronella, lemongrass, palmarosa, vetiver*—these strong aromatic grasses are uplifting, grounding, diuretic, immune and endocrine builders. Just as grasses (grains) are the basis of diet, the grass oils give us bass and body notes for blending.

Labiatae (Mint Family) - *Basil, clary sage, hyssop, lavender, lemon balm, marjoram, patchouli, pennyroyal, peppermint, rosemary, sage, savory, thyme*—all of the mint family are olfactory overachievers. They are adaptogens and medicinal plants without peer. All are aromatics, carminatives, immune stimulants, balancers, mood elevators.

Lauracea (Laurel Family) - *Cassia, bay, camphor, cinnamon, rosewood*—these trees produce oils from their wood, bark, and leaves that are stimulating, bring fire, fluid movement, and create energy enhancement.

Myrtaceae (Myrtle Family) - *Cajeput, clove, eucalyptus, myrtle, niaouli, nutmeg, tea tree*—these trees are so strong that they have no natural enemies (unless you see Koala bears as dangerous—they eat only eucalyptus). Their oils give us inner strength. They are anti-inflammatory, antiseptic, respiratory tract and immune stimulants. In blends they are clean, refreshing, and medicinal.

Rutacea (Citrus Family) - *Bergamot, grapefruit, lemon, lime, mandarin, neroli, orange, petitgrain, tangerine*—this family is known for its fruit and flowers. In blends they are clean and refreshing, uplifting, invigorating, opening, warm, fluid-moving, stimulating, and encouraging. Our life is richer because of citrus.

Umbelliferae (Carrot Family) - *Angelica, ajwan, brahmi, galbanum, anise, caraway, carrot seed, coriander, cumin, dill, fennel, parsley*—rival to the mint family in healing properties, they characteristically reach out with flowers and foliage to embrace the sun and air elements. They are carminative, rejuvenative, stimulant, tonic, regulators of hormones, and useful in skin care.

Zingiberaceae (Ginger Family) - *Cardamon, tumeric, ginger*—these spicy roots bring the fire and earth elements to us. They are grounding, heating, digestive stimulants.

We gratefully acknowledge Drs. David Frawley and Vasant Lad *(Yoga of Herbs)* for their information and organization on the dosha effects, energies, tastes, actions, and tissues of herbs, which we have adapted to essential oil use wherever appropriate.

ANISE

Bryan: While living in Hawaii we often flew between the islands in small commuter planes. On one occasion, after a late start and a quick breakfast, I found myself on a wildly pitching plane in a sudden tropical storm with a very queasy stomach. One frightened person in the back of the plane lost it. The overpowering smell of her stomach contents soon had everyone in the plane pretty close to losing theirs. I fortunately had my kit with me and put a few drops of anise seed oil directly on my tongue, noticed immediate relief, and made it to touchdown without incident. Another happy ending with essential oils.

Anise is very soothing to the nervous stomach, healing to the entire digestive system, and has a detoxifying effect on the liver. Anise is often used as an additive to oriental and middle eastern foods, and is used as a flavoring and an additive to many liquors served in the same region. Anise seed is part of the mixture which is served at the end of an Indian meal to calm digestion. In addition to internal use, it can be massaged onto the abdomen to ease flatulence. Also an excellent expectorant, it can relieve excessive mucous and coughing when administered in a cough syrup. It has aphrodisiac qualities and can be used for frigidity. It is used both internally and externally to relieve cramping.

Common name: Anise

Family name: Umbelliferae (Carrot)

Botanical name: Pimpinella Anisum

Dosha effect: VK–, P+

Taste: pungent

PD taste: pungent

Energy: heating, moisturizing

Actions: carminative, galactagogue, stimulant, diaphoretic

Tissues: stomach, lung, small intestine

Indications: mucous, hard dry cough, gas

Warning: may irritate ulcers, excess use may cause dizziness

Usage: food or drink flavoring, massage oil, compress, inhalations, cough drops

Aroma: intensely sweet, clean, reminiscent of the crushed fruit

Mixes well with: fennel, cardamon, clove

BASIL

There are many varieties of basil. Most common in aromatherapy is the European variety. We also enjoy the Indian variety known as *tulsi* or *basil Krishna*, so named for the story that Krishna always wore garlands of this basil around his neck. He used the Holy basil to produce detachment, faith and devotion. It is known to be one of the sacred plants of India, as it opens the heart and brings harmony to the mind. Basil has strong effects on the emotions, and can be very strengthening when we are suffering fear or sadness. It has many properties that have been very beneficial in asthma and headaches. Basil can be particularly effective when used in a warm compress over the liver and gall bladder.

Common name: Basil Krishna

Family name: Labiatae (Mint)

Botanical name: Ocymum Basilicum

Other name: Tulsi (Indian)

Dosha effect: VK–, P+ in excess

Taste: pungent

PD taste: pungent

Energy: heating, neutral

Actions: diaphoretic, febrifuge (stops fever), nervine, antispasmodic, antibacterial, antiseptic, cephalic (clears congestion in the head), emmenagogue, antifungal

Tissues: plasma, blood, marrow and nerves, reproductive organs, liver, lungs

Indications: colds, cough, sinus congestion, headaches, arthritis, rheumatism, fevers (generally), abdominal conditions, pregnancy, nursing, asthma, and poor clarity of mind

Warning: avoid use in high Pitta condition, pregnancy

Usage: tea, juice, medicated ghee, cooking, inhalation, compress, aroma lamp

Aroma: sweet-spicy, slightly green, fresh, with faint balsamic-woody undertone and a lasting sweetness

Mixes well with: camphor, rosemary, juniper, lemon, eucalyptus, myrtle, lavender, opoponox, bergamot, clary sage, lime, oak moss

BAY

There are two species of plants distilled in two different parts of the world and sold under the name bay. The bay from Europe is in the laurel family. The bay from the West Indies is in the myrtle family. Fortunately, they have many similar properties. One of Light's favorite uses is to add bay to hot oil treatment for the hair. To two ounces of jojoba oil, add 4 drops of bay, 3 drops of lavender, 3 drops of lemon, 3 drops of rosemary, 3 drops of rosewood, and a tablespoon of sesame oil. Heat the mixture and apply to the hair while warm, wrap your head in a towel, and sit for fifteen minutes to half an hour. Shampoo clean. Bay is also very effective for dry scalp and hair; you may add it to shampoo and cream rinses. Several drops in a water solution can stimulate nail growth and strength. Bay can be useful for the respiratory tract, also easing congestion or colds, especially in combination with eucalyptus and rosemary.

Common name: Bay

Family Name: Laurus Nobilis (Laurel family)

Botanical name: Pimenta Racemosa Myrtaceae-Myrtle

Dosha effect: V K P+

Taste: pungent, bitter, astringent

PD taste: pungent

Energy: heating, drying

Actions: stimulant, expectorant, antiseptic, analgesic, carminative, antineuralgic

Tissues: hair, nails, stomach, small intestine

Indications: respiratory problems, infectious diseases, muscular & anticular pain, neuralgia, scalp dryness

Warning: in excess, can cause cramping

Usage: food, lotion, oil treatment, massage oil, compress

Aroma: fresh, spicy, somewhat medicinal, a lasting, sweet-balsamic undertone (sickly sweet, nauseating to some people)

Mixes well with: lavender, eucalyptus, lemon, rosemary, petitgrain, geranium, citronella, cinnamon and ylang ylang

BENZOIN

Benzoin is excellent for use in perfume mixtures because it is a fixative and will hold on to the lighter notes, and because it is a preservative and will prevent oils from becoming oxidized. It is very beneficial to an irritated nervous system and can be useful in depression, PMS, and stress. Externally it can be used to promote the healing of wounds. Used by estheticians for dry, irritated skin and to soften scars.

Common name: Benzoin

Family name: Styracae (Styrax)

Botanical name: Styrax Benzoin

Dosha effect: V P K–

Taste: sweet, bitter, pungent

PD taste: sweet

Energy: heating, moisturizing

Actions: nervine, diuretic, balancing, antiseptic, expectorant, anti-inflammatory, preservative

Tissues: skin, nerves, respiratory, urinary, hormonal

Indications: nervous conditions, depression, PMS, irritability, stress, throat infection, coughs, bronchitis, asthma, dry cough, irritated skin, circulation, genito-urinary infections, skin cuts and infections

Warning: none

Usage: compress, perfumes, massage oils, salve

Aroma: pleasant, sweet-balsamic with distinct note of vanillin

Mixes well with: almost any oil, especially as a fixative and preservative

BERGAMOT

Bryan: Bergamot is a wonderful antidepressant. One of our sons was having difficulty in his senior year of High School. He was experiencing severe depression, in part due to the fact that upon graduation we were going on the road to travel and teach, and he would no longer have a home. We got a call from his teachers stating that he had been absent sixty-five days, and for the remainder of the school year he would have to go to school on weekends in order to graduate. They warned that although his grades were good, he must have perfect attendance for the last month of school. Knowing the rebellious nature of teenagers, Light began to sneak into his room every morning and put a few drops of bergamot and lemongrass on his pillow as he slept. We noticed an immediate change. He would get up on time, take a bath, eat a hearty breakfast, call his friends and arrange a ride to school, speak animatedly and excitedly at the breakfast table about his coming day. It was a miraculous transformation. This was the child who only days before was difficult to wake up, grumpy, uncommunicative. After a week of this he came to us and said, "What are you guys doing to me? My room smells like herbs." When we explained how we were medicating him he said, "Just give me the oils and I'll take a bath in the morning, I do feel better." And he did, and he graduated and the rest is history.

We find that people who suffer depression are unable to experience and enjoy the richness of life, which reflects itself in liver congestion and gall bladder obstruction. Bergamot can be used in a compress directly over the liver and gall bladder. Bergamot is made from the skin of a citrus fruit that is grown almost exclusively in the southern tip of Italy and a few places in the Mediterranean.

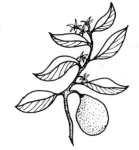

The bergamot essential oil is mainly cold pressed. Sometimes it is sold BF (bergaptene free) for more gentle use on the skin. It is also possible to buy steam distilled bergamot essential oil which is the treatment of choice for skin, but very expensive. Because many of the components of bergamot oil are filtered through the urinary tract, it can be very useful in kidney and bladder infections. It is excellent for addictions. Taken orally, it also helps to calm the digestion. Bergamot is well known for its use in Earl Gray tea. Externally, it is very effective in working with skin irritations. It can help reduce fevers. I like adding it to pancake batter for an unusual lemon-like taste.

BERGAMOT (continued)

Common name: Bergamot

Family name: Rutacea

Botanical name: Citrus Bergamia

Dosha effect: V K–, P+

Taste: sweet, sour, astringent

PD taste: pungent

Energy: heating, drying

Actions: antiseptic, antipyretic, antidepressant, vulnerary, antispasmodic, astringent, appetite stimulant

Tissues: all elements

Indications: gingivitis, sore throat, cystitis, vaginal itching (discharge), fungus, fever, lost appetite, colic, flatulence, intestinal parasites, emotional imbalance, acne, psoriasis, eczema, bladder infection

Warning: do not apply oil to skin in greater than a .5 to 1% diluted form in base oil

Usage: tea, mouthwash, compress, aroma lamp, lotion, perfumes, massage oil, bath, inhalation

Aroma: rich, sweet-fruity initial odor, followed by a still more characteristic oily-herbaceous and somewhat balsamic body and dryout; the sweetness yields to a more tobacco-like and rich note, somewhat reminiscent of clary sage and neryl-acetate

Mixes well with: cypress, jasmine, juniper, lavender, neroli, lemongrass, all citrus

BIRCH

The sap of the birch tree is collected in the same way as the maple; collected in buckets and boiled into a syrup. It has historically been used to make birch or root beer. Its bark is often distilled with wintergreen leaves and birch oil has often been substituted for wintergreen. It is sometimes used in after-shave lotions because it has a smell reminiscent of leather. Its most therapeutic uses involve external application, especially for sore, cramped muscles, and for skin or scalp irritations. It is excellent as an addition to shampoos because it promotes hair growth. A recipe for stimulating hair growth, a hot oil treatment for hair loss: into one ounce of coconut oil add five drops of chamomile, five drops of coriander, and five drops of birch. Massage the oil into your scalp before you shampoo. Allow fifteen minutes to soak in.

Common name: Birch

Family name: Betulacea

Botanical name: Betula Lenulta

Dosha effect: P K–, V+

Taste: bitter, pungent

PD taste: pungent

Energy: cooling, moisturizing

Actions: diaphoretic, diuretic, analgesic, astringent, dissolves uric acid, alterative

Tissues: joints, muscle, scalp, kidneys, skin

Indications: rheumatism, wounds, sore or cramped muscles, tendinitis, skin rashes, ulcers, cellulite, toxin & fluid accumulation

Warning: do not use if excess Vata, underweight

Usage: bath, massage oil, compresses, treatment for hair loss

Aroma: (bark) strikingly similar to methyl salicylate, (bud) pleasant woody-green, balsamic odor

Mixes well with: wintergreen, eucalyptus, myrtle, juniper, orange, lavender, pine, fir, rosemary

BLACK PEPPER

Black pepper oil can be used in a formula for weight loss. Recipe: 10 drops lavender, 5 drops frankincense, 5 drops sandalwood, and 10 drops black pepper oil in three ounces of mustard, canola, almond oil, or a mixture. To be used externally on areas where you wish to lose weight. As a carminative it can be added to foods. Occasionally used in blends for energetic enhancement. Used for toothache (direct application) and externally for joint and muscle aching.

Common name: Black Pepper

Family name: Piperaseae

Botanical name: Piper Nigrum

Other name: Marich (sanskrit name for sun), as it contains large amounts of solar

Energy: heating, drying

Dosha effect: K–, P V+ (in excess)

Taste: pungent, bitter

PD taste: pungent

Energy: heating, drying

Actions: stimulant, expectorant, carminative, febrifuge, anthelmintic, diuretic

Tissues: plasma, blood, fat, marrow, nerve, spleen, urinary tract, digestive

Indications: chronic indigestion, toxins in colon, degenerated metabolism, obesity, sinus congestion, intermittent fever, cold extremities

Warning: do not use with inflammatory conditions of the digestive organs, high Pitta

Usage: weight reduction, cooking, lotion, compress

Aroma: fresh, dry-woody, warm-spicy, reminiscent of dried black pepper and elemi, cubeb and other high terpene-sesquiterpene oils

Mixes well with: orange, cypress, ginger, ajwan, birch, anise seed, rose, sandalwood, frankincense, lemon, basil

CAJEPUT

Cajeput oil is an excellent hemostatic. While traveling in the western United States, a friend of Light's severely cut the tip of her finger. People who saw the wound said that it *had* to be stitched. Light immediately put Cajeput oil in and on the wound, held it together, and then secured it with a Band-Aid®. The wound healed nicely in three to four days.

In the same family as tea tree, this oil is highly antiseptic. Its smell, which is similar to eucalyptus, can be useful in inhalations for bronchial conditions. It can be used in a gargle with sandalwood oil for sore throat; recipe: 1 drop cajeput, 1 drop sandalwood in one half cup water, mix well and gargle. This has been used with success by many singers who have lost their voice through a combination of stress and colds. Cajeput is most effective when massaged around the voice box to alleviate the associated muscle tension. It is excellent for joint and muscle distress as it blends well with eucalyptus, rosemary, juniper, and camphor as a liniment, very strong massage oil or compress.

While taking a tour group through cities like Bombay and Calcutta, Light soaked handkerchiefs in a combination of cajeput and lemon, and had the group wear these kerchiefs over their nose and mouth to prevent irritation and infection. No one in the tour group got sick.

Common name: Cajeput

Family name: Myrtaceae

Botanical name: Melaleuca Leuadendrom

Other name: Katupruhi [Indian name]

Dosha effect: K V–, P+

Taste: bitter, pungent, sweet

PD taste: pungent

Energy: heating, moisturizing

Actions: antiseptic, antispasmodic, expectorant, analgesic, antineuralgic, hemostatic

Tissues: skin, epithelial

Indications: colds, throat diseases, pains, headaches, bronchitis, diarrhea, urinary tract infections, stomach cramps, inflammation of small intestine, nervous vomiting, intestinal parasites, rheumatism, neuralgia, earaches, toothaches, psoriasis, acne

Warning: in high dosage may cause vomiting and stomach irritation

Usage: throat lozenges, gargles, ear oil

CAJEPUT (continued)

Aroma: powerful, fresh, eucalyptus-like, camphoraceous odor, almost fruity-sweet body notes and soft tones in the dryout

Mixes well with: eucalyptus, rosemary, camphor, juniper, cypress, tea tree

CALAMUS

Calamus strengthens the adrenals. It is useful in periods of weakness, beneficial for gingivitis, can be a stimulant to lymphatic drainage; provides relief in extreme back pain. It has a very strong and somewhat unpleasant odor, which is reminiscent of male goat. Fortunately, this can be overcome by using sweeter oils like lavender. It increases endurance and stamina. This is an oil we recommend to use only externally. Calamus does contain components that are known carcinogens. While thousands of years of herbal use in India have demonstrated its clinical effectiveness and safety, we recommend *no* internal use of this essential oil.

Common name: Calamus Sweet Flag

Family name: Acorus Calumus (Araceae family)

Dosha effect: V K–, P+

Taste: pungent, bitter, astringent

PD taste: pungent

Energy: heating/drying

Actions: stimulant, rejuvenative, expectorant, decongestant, nervine, antispasmodic, emetic

Tissues: plasma, muscle, fat, marrow and nerve, reproductive

Systems: nervous, respiratory, digestive, circulatory, reproductive

Indications: colds, cough, asthma, sinus headaches, sinusitis, arthritis, epilepsy, shock, coma, loss of memory, deafness, hysteria, neuralgia

Warning: not recommended for internal use, can cause bleeding disorders, including nose bleeds and hemorrhoids

Usage: externally in compress or massage oil

Aroma: warm woody-spice and pleasant odor with increasingly sweet aftertones and great tenacity

Mixes well with: lavender and ginger, lemon and orange, yarrow, eucalyptus, myrtle, birch, cinnamon, labdanum, olibanum, patchouli and cedarwood

CAMPHOR

Camphor can be produced synthetically, so it is important to make sure that the camphor you are purchasing is from natural sources and is steam distilled. Also, when camphor is steam distilled it is fractionalized. The fractions are named white, brown and blue. Blue camphor is the heaviest, consisting mainly of sesquiterpenes and sesquiterpene alcohols of weak odor; used in perfume as a fixative; not readily available. Brown camphor contains up to 80% safrole, which is a known carcinogen and should be avoided at all costs. White camphor is more commonly sold. This is the oil that is used for medicinal purposes in China, Japan and India. Camphor increases prana, opens up senses and brings clarity to the mind, eases headache and awakens perception. It is a good stimulant and counter-irritant for joint and muscle pain. In excess, camphor acts as a narcotic poison, aggravating Pitta and Vata.

Common name: Camphor
Family name: Cinnamomum Camphora or Champora Officinarum
Botanical name: Lauraceae (Laurel)
Other name: Karpura(s)
Dosha effect: K V–, P+ (in excess)
Taste: pungent, sour
PD taste: pungent
Energy: heating, moisturizing
Actions: expectorant, decongestant, stimulant, antispasmodic, bronchodilator, nervine, analgesic, antiseptic
Tissues: plasma, blood, fat, marrow, nerve
Systems: respiratory, nervous
Indications: bronchitis, asthma, whooping cough, pulmonary congestion, hysteria, epilepsy, delirium, insomnia, dysmenorrhea, gout, rheumatism, nasal congestion, sinus headaches, eye problems, tooth decay
Warning: use only in low dosage (3-5 drops per oz. of vegetable oil)
Usage: massage oil, compress, salve, inhalation diffuser, lotions
Aroma: strong, sharp, bitter, medicinal
Mixes well with: rosemary, eucalyptus, frankincense, juniper, wintergreen

CARAWAY

Caraway is traditionally used in European baking as an additive to bread, to aid in the assimilation of starch. This was also practiced in ancient Egypt. It is known to reduce gas (flatulence). It's not commonly used in aroma therapy. The oil is used in India for parasites in a basti (enema). Can also help mental clarity and alertness.

Common name: Caraway

Family name: Umbelliferae (Carrot)

Botanical name: Carum Carvi

Dosha effect: K V–, P+

Taste: pungent

PD taste: pungent

Energy: heating/drying

Actions: carminative, stimulant, depurative, antispasmodic

Tissues: digestive, scalp

Indications: indigestion, gas, colic, nervous conditions, accumulation (toxins, fluids)

Warning: can make skin more sensitive to sunlight

Usage: cooking, perfumes in very diluted %, "tummy rub" for gas

Aroma: (crude) strong and peculiar odor typical of the fruit, with a fatty-harsh undertone, initial note of nauseating, almost amine-like type (rectified) stronger, less fatty.

Mixes well with: dill, fennel, anise, basil, jasmine

CARDAMON

Cardamon stimulates the mind and heart and brings clarity and joy. Added to milk it neutralizes its mucous-forming properties and detoxifies caffeine in coffee. Its quality is sattvic and it is particularly good for opening and soothing the flow of the pranas in the body. It helps stop vomiting, belching, or acid regurgitation. Cardamon is good for the nervous digestive upset of children or of high Vata. Helps digest fats and starches, stimulates the spleen, opens the heart, brings mind clarity and stability, joy, and festivity. Antidote to caffeine, excellent for low digestive fire. Good for Vata because it kindles agni (fire). Removes excess Kapha from the stomach and lungs.

Name:	Cardamon
Family name:	Ziniberaceae (Ginger)
Botanical name:	Eletarria Cardamomom
Dosha effect:	V K–, P+ in excess
Taste:	pungent/sweet
PD taste:	pungent
Energy:	heating, moisturizing
Actions:	stimulant, expectorant, carminative, stomachic, diaphoretic, aphrodisiac
Tissues:	plasma, blood, marrow and nerve
Indications:	colds, cough, bronchitis, asthma, hoarse voice, loss of taste, poor absorption, indigestion, impotence
Warning:	do not use with ulcers, high Pitta
Usage:	tea, coffee, aroma lamp, perfume, massage oil, bath, food
Aroma:	warm spicy, aromatic with a balsamic floral undertone
Mixes well with:	orange, anise, rose, bergamot, caraway, ginger, shamama, jatamansi, olibanum, ylang ylang, labdanum, neroli, cedarwood and coriander

CARROT SEED

Carrot seed comes in a cold-pressed form and also a steam-distilled form, which is more expensive. It has many uses in skin care. It tones and tightens. It is especially good to repair aging or damaged skin. Effective when experiencing feelings of separation, fogginess, and dizziness.

Common name: Carrot Seed

Family name: Umbelliferae

Botanical name: Daucus Carota

Dosha effect: V P K=

Taste: sweet, pungent

PD Taste: sweet

Energy: heating and moisturizing

Actions: increases tanning, tonic, depurative, stimulates elasticity, helps nourish, tighten, revitalize and rejuvenate skin, stimulates lymph system, aids women's milk production

Tissues: skin, lymphatic, liver system, GI tract

Indications: abscesses, boils, ulcers, skin disorders, liver and gall bladder disorders, hepatitis, colitis, enteritis

Warning: over exposure to sun may cause discoloration

Usage: spice blends, seasonings, skin lotion, masks, food and drink

Aroma: peculiar dry-woody, somewhat root-like, earthy odor; the initial notes are sweet and fresh, but tenacious undertone and dryout is very heavy, sweet-earthy, fatty-oily, slightly spicy

Mixes well with: geranium, lavender, rose, dhavana, sandalwood, jatamansi, vetiver, citrus oils, cedarwood

CEDARWOOD

This oil is from the juniper family and is quite different from Himalayan cedar. It is the smell we associate with cedar chests, and this oil is reasonably priced so you can purchase it by the ounce and use it to put that "cedar" smell back in cedar wood. Originally the wood was used in construction because it was a repellent to moths and other insects that consumed clothes. It is very useful for discouraging any insects, including mosquitos and fleas. Cedar should be avoided during pregnancy as a possible abortifactant. This fragrance is wonderful for cleansing the atmosphere in a room; also a disinfectant for urinary tract infections, but should be avoided in acute kidney infections; wonderful for sore joints and muscles; has multiple uses for oily skin and acne; and will help provoke an overdue menstrual cycle.

Common name: Cedarwood

Family name: Pinaceae (Pine)

Botanical name: Juniperus Virginiana

Dosha effect: P, K–, V+

Taste: bitter, sweet, pungent

PD taste: pungent

Energy: heating, drying

Actions: antiseptic, expectorant, diuretic, nervine, rejuvenating

Tissues: urinary, skin, scalp

Indications: bronchitis, urinary infections, fear, nervous tension, aggression, psychological disconnectedness, oily hair, hair loss

Warning: contains thujon, should not be taken orally in high doses, not to be taken when pregnant; can irritate central nervous system, burn stomach lining, and cause severe thirst

Usage: soap perfumery, mosquito-repellent, disinfectant, insecticide, cleansers, compresses, teas, baths, massage oil, inhalations

Aroma: at first, oily, mild and pleasant, somewhat balsamic, the odor becomes drier, more woody, less balsamic as oil dries

Mixes well with: juniper, camphor, eucalyptus, sandalwood, patchouli, vetiver, citronella

HIMALAYAN CEDARWOOD

I prefer Himalayan cedarwood to the Virginia cedar. Grown at high altitude in the Himalayas, it has a sweet, rich top note which gives a sense of clarity and connectedness. Whereas Virginia cedarwood is in the juniper family, Himalayan cedarwood is a true "cedar," closer to the Cedars of Lebanon. It continues to have excellent healing properties in cases of infection of the kidneys and urinary tract. This oil is calming and elevating, an anti-depressive, very helpful in breathing problems, especially bronchial congestion. Spiritually, it can be used when developing or mastering a pranayama (breathing exercise).

Common name: Cedarwood, Himalayan
Family name: Pinaceae
Botanical name: Ceodora Deodara
Dosha effect: V P K=
Taste: sweet, bitter, pungent
PD taste: pungent
Energy: heating, drying
Actions: antiseptic, expectorant, diuretic, nervine, rejuvenative
Tissues: endocrine system, nerve, respiratory, urinary tract
Indications: headache, urinary infection, arthritis
Warning: do not take internally during pregnancy
Usage: soap, aftershave, massage oil, meditation, bath
Aroma: rich, sweet-woody, almost balsamic odor, has camphoraceous top-notes, but delicately sweet-woody on its lasting dryout.
Mixes well with: jatamansi, sandalwood, pine, dhavana, labdanum, petitgrain, rosewood, calamus, clary sage, vetiver and ylang ylang

BLUE CHAMOMILE

Light: Blue chamomile, along with rose, lavender, and geranium, are some of the few oils that can be used directly on the skin, in small amounts, in part due to their mild, neutral nature, and in part due to the oil on your skin (your natural body oil). When you rub one drop of blue chamomile onto an external bruise, it blends with your natural skin oil and is especially potent and effective. A favorite for burns, fevers and skin irritation, it also has extensive internal use due to its immune building and anti-inflammatory properties. When my niece had chicken pox, my sister-in-law put a drop in every one of the spots, and within two days the child was clear.

Common name: Chamomile, Blue (German)

Family name: Compositae (Sunflower)

Botanical name: Matricaria Chamomilla

Dosha effect: P V–, K+ (in excess)

Taste: sweet, bitter

PD Taste: sweet

Energy: cooling/drying

Actions: anti-inflammatory, immuno-stimulant, analgesic, antispasmodic, sedative, emmenagogue, antianemic, digestive, cholagogue, hepatic

Tissues: skin, all tissues

Indications: dermatitis, inflamed skin, leukocyte formation, arthritis, abscess, colic, colitis, headache, insomnia, irritability, amenorrhea, dysmenorrhea, menopause, teething, toothache, anemia, digestive problems, liver/spleen congestion, feminine reproductive problems, anger, tantrum, burns

Warning: none

Usage: massage oil, skin lotion, aroma lamp, inhalation, baths, food and drink

Aroma: intensely sweet, herbaceous-coumarin-like odor with a fresh-fruity undertone; dryout is pleasant sweet tobacco-like and warm (of mellow and aged oil); freshly distilled, an obnoxiously animal-sweet, amine-like note

Mixes well with: lavender, cajeput, tea tree, rose, yarrow, angelica, calamus, bergamot, cardamon, sandalwood, geranium

GOLD CHAMOMILE

This is the chamomile that is preferred for children's illnesses because of its soothing and calming effect. It's closer to the central part of the chart than the blue chamomile. It is excellent for babies when their gums are irritated from teething. Inhalation works well for tension, stress and irritability. This holds true for adults too. It can be of special assistance during menopause and PMS. Also similar in properties to Roman chamomile, a domestic variety available in the United States, which is of good quality and more affordable.

Common name: Chamomile (Roman)

Family name: Compositae (Sunflower)

Botanical name: Anthemis Nobilis

Dosha effect: K P–, V+ (in excess)

Taste: bitter, pungent, sweet

PD taste: sweet

Energy: cooling/neutral

Actions: diaphoretic, antipyretic, anti-inflammatory, carminative, nervine, antispasmodic, analgesic, emmenagogue, emetic

Tissues: plasma, blood, muscles, marrow, nerve

Indications: headaches, indigestion, nervous problems in children, colic, eye inflammations, jaundice, dysmenorrhea, amenorrhea, insomnia, anger, depression, PMS, sunburn

Warning: large dosages are emetic and may aggravate Vata

Usage: all uses are good

Aroma: sweet herbaceous, somewhat fruity-warm and tealeaf-like odor, extremely diffusive, little tenacity, fresh herbal smell.

Mixes well with: rose, lavender, ylang ylang, cedar, geranium, tangerine, fennel, cinnamon, jasmine, bergamot, neroli, clary sage, labdanum, oakmoss

MOROCCAN CHAMOMILE

Moroccan chamomile is actually a member of the tansy family, gathered wild on the hillsides of Morocco. When distilled, azulene is produced, and makes this oil a very deep blue color. Its smell is much warmer and sweeter than the somewhat bitter blue chamomile. Having many of the same medicinal properties, it finds wider use in perfumery because of its sweetness.

Common name: Chamomile (Moroccan)

Family name: Tanacetum Annum

Botanical name: Ormenis Multicaulis

Dosha effect: V P–, K+ (in excess)

Taste: sweet, bitter, pungent

PD taste: sweet

Energy: cooling, drying

Actions: anti-inflammatory, analgesic, antispasmodic, sedative, cholagogue, hepatic

Tissues: skin

Indications: acne, dermatitis, inflamed skin, arthritis, abscess, bruises, colic (external application)

Warning: external use only if absolute

Usage: massage oil, skin lotion, shampoo, conditioner

Aroma: intensely sweet, warm like fresh-mown hay with floral undertones

Mixes well with: rose, lavender, chamomile, geranium, jatamansi, juniper, cypress, labdanum, vetiver, cedarwood

CINNAMON

Light: Cinnamon is one of the best oils for circulation, especially during menopause. It improves sexual function, increases sexual desire, and improves digestion and appetite. Because it enhances circulation, it is very supportive of the heart. It is empowering to the will. Cinnamon can be useful for parasites, scabies, or lice. Cinnamon bark oil has a high percentage of aldehyde and is not recommended for use on the skin as it can be irritating. Cinnamon leaf oil has a very low percentage of aldehyde and is more suitable for use in liniments or massage oils. When I wake up on a cold morning, sometimes feeling sluggish, I add a few drops of cinnamon oil to my sesame oil, to help get me going.

Common name: Cinnamon

Family name: Lauraceae (Laurel)

Botanical name: Cinnamomum Zeylanicum

Other name: Twak(s) Indian

Dosha effect: V K–, P+

Taste: pungent, sweet, astringent

PD taste: sweet

Energy: heating/neutral

Actions: stimulant, diaphoretic, parasiticide, aphrodisiac, antispasmodic, expectorant, analgesic, diuretic, alterative, carminative

Tissues: plasma, blood, muscle, marrow and nerves

Indications: colds, sinus congestion, bronchitis, dyspepsia, circulation, spasms, anemia, asthenia, lice, scabies, impotence, childbirth, intestinal infections, menopause

Warning: do not use in condition of high Pitta; will aggravate bleeding disorders; skin irritant in high dose; convulsive in high doses

Usage: food, drink, massage oil, aroma lamp, liniment

Aroma: (bark)extremely powerful, diffusive, warm-spicy, sweet and tenacious odor; (leaf) warm-spicy, but rather harsh odor, lacking rich body of bark oil. Some resemblance to clove leaf and clove stem oil

Mixes well with: cardamon, orange, nutmeg, anise, fennel, trifolia

CITRONELLA

Bryan: Never go camping without citronella; it is a wonderful mosquito and insect repellent. I use it when I shampoo my dog's hair; 20 drops of citronella added to two tablespoons of shampoo is very effective at killing fleas. Just wet your pet down, massage in the shampoo and citronella mix, let stand for five minutes, and rinse away. Your dog might not like the bath but he may enjoy the massage you give him as you work the suds into his coat. After you have dried him off and he has attacked the towel and worked off his aggression, he will smell great. He will be a happy dog with no fleas.

Common name:	Citronella
Family name:	Graminae (Grass)
Botanical name:	Cymbopagon Nardus
Dosha effect:	P K–, V
Taste:	bitter, sweet
PD taste:	pungent
Energy:	warming, moisturizing
Actions:	mosquito repellent, flea repellent, deodorizer, purifier, stimulant, antiseptic
Tissues:	skin
Indications:	digestive problems and infectious diseases
Warning:	do not take internally (due to aldehyde content)
Usage:	apply oil to skin or pet's fur, aroma lamp, spritzer, diffuser, insect repellent
Aroma:	(Ceylon) very peculiar, warm-woody and yet fresh, grassy and somewhat reminiscent of wet leaves; camphene-borneol-methyleugenol complex is characteristic of odor; (Java-type) fresh and sweet, dryout is sweet, somewhat woody
Mixes well with:	lemon, eucalyptus, lavender, pennyroyal, geranium, rose, cedarwood

CLARY SAGE

Clary sage is a gift to the female; no woman should ever be without it. It gives women a sense of clarity and empowerment, helping to get rid of monthly bloat, depression, and anxiety, regulating menses, and cooling down hot flashes. It is a gift to the Goddess. In addition to its relaxing and cramp-relieving properties, it is known to be euphoric, and at one time was added to German beer and wine. Clary sage has a rejuvenating effect on the endocrine system. It balances the pituitary and has many of the beneficial effects of sage without having sage's toxicity. It is a special friend for the woman going through menopause and can not only be used internally, but it is especially effective at feeding estrogen directly into the skin.

Phillip Morris is a large producer of clary sage. They grow the clary sage on a farm in North Carolina. They harvest it in such a way that it goes directly into the stainless steel tank of a truck; the truck pulls up to the distillery, and super-heated steam is forced through the tank, through the clary sage. The volatile components are carried through pipes back into the factory. The super-heated steam is then condensed and the clary sage is condensed out. The truck with the spent clary sage then goes back to the field to dispose of the used herbal matter. A very efficient operation.

Common name:	Clary Sage
Family name:	Labiatae
Botanical name:	Salvia Sclarea
Dosha effect:	V P K–
Taste:	sweet, bitter, pungent
PD taste:	pungent
Energy:	warming/neutral
Actions:	digestive stimulant, stomachic, nervine, antispasmodic, aphrodisiac, antiseptic, deodorizing
Tissues:	skin, nerve, reproductive
Indications:	cramps, weak digestion, flatulence, bronchitis, asthma, PMS, childbirth, headache, psychological tension, nerves, fear, impotence, frigidity, infected skin, swollen tissue
Warning:	do not combine with alcohol, or take orally with any medication containing iron
Usage:	all uses are good

CLARY SAGE (continued)

Aroma: sweet, herbaceous, tenacious; soft, somewhat reminiscent of ambra in its bittersweet undertone, dryout odor is tobacco-like; some call it balsamic or tea-like

Mixes well with: geranium, lavender, jatamansi, yarrow, vetiver, bergamot, labdanum, olibanum, cinnamon, rosewood, coriander, cardamon, citrus oils, cedarwood

CLOVE

Clove is one of the oldest essential oils. Traditionally used for toothaches, it is approved by the American Dental Association as an anesthetic. Because it is very strengthening to the musculature, it has been traditionally recommended that expectant mothers consume cloves in the last month of pregnancy to tone the uterus and prepare it for the birth process. Tantrics have recommended a mild dilution of clove oil to decrease the male sensitivity, as an aid in premature ejaculation.

Common name:	Clove Bud
Family name:	Myrtaceae (Myrtle)
Botanical name:	Eugenia Caryophyllata
Other name:	Lavanga
Dosha effect:	K V–, P+
Taste:	pungent
PD taste:	pungent
Energy:	heating
Actions:	stimulant, carminative, aphrodisiac, expectorant, analgesic
Tissues:	plasma, muscle, marrow and nerve, reproductive
Indications:	colds, cough, asthma, indigestion, toothache, vomiting, hiccough, laryngitis, pharyngitis, low blood pressure, impotence
Warning:	don't use if inflammatory condition, hypertension, or high Pitta is present
Usage:	skin, compress, perfume, aroma lamp, massage oil, lotion, food and drink
Aroma:	a peculiar fruity-fresh topnote, acetic odor quite refreshing, with a sweet spicy note.
Mixes well with:	cardamon, cinnamon, lavender, ginger, orange, vanilla, rose, clary sage, bergamot, bay leaf, ylang ylang

CORIANDER

This fresh green herb is also known as cilantro or Chinese parsley, and is a favorite in Mexican food. The essential oil is produced from the seed, is an antidote to hot food, very decongesting to the liver, and is a great reducer of fire and heat in the body. It is thought to be an aphrodisiac because of its phyto-estrogen content. It's also a carminative, stimulating digestion.

Common name: Coriander

Family name: Umbelliferae (Carrot)

Botanical name: Coriandrum Sativum

Other name: Dhanyaka

Dosha effect: V P K–

Taste: bitter, pungent, sweet

PD taste: pungent

Energy: cooling/moisturizing

Actions: alterative, diaphoretic, diuretic, carminative, stimulant

Tissues: plasma, blood, muscle

Indications: burning urethra, cystitis, urinary tract infection, urticaria, rash, burns, sore throat, vomiting, indigestion, allergies, hay fever

Warning: few warnings, except high Vata with nerve tissue deficiency; may cause kidney irritation in high dose, do not take during pregnancy

Usage: cooking, compresses, douche, patch, massage oil, shampoo

Aroma: pleasant, sweet, somewhat woody-spicy aromatic-candy like odor, floral-balsamic undertone; peppery-woody, suave topnote

Mixes well with: lemon, tea tree, cajaput, lavender, peppermint, cardamon, bergamot, clove, clary sage, nutmeg, jasmine, petitgrain, sandalwood, cypress

CUBEB

This herb has a light peppery smell. On occasion, when substituted into a formula for weight loss instead of black pepper, patients reported greater effectiveness. In *The Aromatherapy Book*, Jenny Rose reports that cubeb stimulates the parathyroid, and so it would be an excellent addition to menopausal formulas, helping with problems of osteoporosis.

Common name:	Cubeb
Family name:	Lauracea (Laurel)
Botanical name:	Piper Cubeb
Dosha effect:	V K–, P+
Taste:	pungent
PD taste:	pungent
Energy:	heating
Actions:	stimulant, carminative, expectorant
Tissues:	blood, plasma
Indications:	digestion, diuretic, skin irritation, weight loss
Warning:	do not use in conditions of high Pitta, do not use directly on skin - always dilute
Usage:	lotions, compresses, bath, perfume-blending
Aroma:	very dry-woody, but simultaneously warm-camphoraceous, spicy-peppery
Mixes well with:	lavender, black pepper, cardamon, cinnamon, anise, clove, galbanum, rosemary

CUMIN

Cumin is one of those essential oils that new aromatherapists are not crazy about because its overpowering smell can ruin any blend if not sufficiently diluted. It is a common flavoring in Mexican and Middle Eastern food. Very small additions to a blend will give erotic character. As a carminative, it is excellent for absorption of nutrients. In California, it's now being used with AIDS patients in building the immune system. We have had success using it to build the immune system of allergy patients.

Common name: Cumin

Family name: Umbelliferae (carrot)

Botanical name: Cuminum Cyminum

Dosha effect: K P–, V+

Taste: pungent, bitter

PD taste: pungent

Energy: cooling/neutral

Actions: carminative, alterative, stimulant, antispasmodic, lactagogue, immune builder

Tissues: heart and uterus, digestive, nerves, muscle

Indications: gas, low breast milk, digestion, nerves, circulation, anemia, convalescence, migraine

Warning: excess may cause nausea

Usage: massage oil, perfumes, compress, food and drink

Aroma: extremely powerful, diffusive, green-spicy, slightly fatty, but not sharp or pungent, almost soft and mellow.

Mixes well with: (in trace amounts) angelica, lemon, black pepper, coriander, lavender, rosemary, rosewood, oakmoss

CYPRESS

Cypress is good for anything in excess due to its astringent properties. It is one of the best oils for Vata because of its grounding nature. We've used it for cuts, hemorrhoids, and excess bleeding. It is a wonderful essential oil for any circulation problems. It has also been used in weight reduction formulas because of its diuretic effect. It is a balancer to the female system, often combined with clary sage for hot flashes and used to reduce or inhibit the growth of ovarian cysts. Because of its work with acne and oily skin it is often added to skin care formulas. Cypress is excellent in aftershave and hair care formulas.

Common name: Cypress

Family name: Cupressaceae

Botanical name: Cupressus Sempervirens

Dosha effect: V K P+

Taste: pungent, sweet, astringent

PD taste: pungent

Energy: warming, drying

Actions: astringent, antispasmodic, expectorant, antiseptic, regulates female hormone system, deodorizing

Tissues: skin, nerves, muscle, scalp

Indications: weak connective tissue, diarrhea, heavy menstruation, bleeding, hemorrhoids, varicose veins, bleeding gums, convulsive and whooping coughs, severe foot perspiration, menopausal problems, ovarian cysts, absent-mindedness, lack of concentration, nervous/emotional breakdown, sexual preoccupation, oily skin, acne, oily hair, dandruff

Warning: do not use directly on the skin, always dilute

Usage: massage oil, patches, compress, lotion, poultices, shampoos, baths, inhalations

Aroma: sweet-balsamic, yet refreshing odor, reminiscent of pine needles, templin oil (European silver fir), juniperberry oil, cardamon oil (without the cineole-note) and a unique dryout of delicate and tenacious sweetness.

Mixes well with: lemon, juniper, birch, bergamot, orange, grapefruit, clary sage, musk, mandarin, Moroccan chamomile, styrax, jasmine

DILL

Dill is not one of the most common oils used in aromatherapy, but it is wonderful as a carminative, food flavoring, and additive to soups and salad dressings. In the carrot family, it has many similar properties to fennel. It promotes the flow of milk, and it helps to regulate or suppress sexual impulses.

Common name: Dill

Family name: Umbelliferae (Carrot)

Botanical Name: Anethum Graveolens

Dosha effect: P K–, V o

Taste: pungent, bitter

PD taste: pungent

Energy: cooling/neutral

Actions: carminative, alterative, nervine, stimulant (digestive), expectorant, antispasmodic, promotes milk flow

Tissues: blood, fat, digestive

Indications: oversexed, flatulence, parasites, nervous vomiting, hiccups

Warning: may decrease sexual energy, cause stinging, reddened or blistered skin, or make skin more sensitive to sunlight

Usage: food (salad dressing), perfumes, massage oil

Aroma: (seed oil) light and fresh, warm-spicy and reminiscent of caraway and spearmint; (weed oil) powerful and fresh, sweet-spicy, peppery and aromatic odor, reminiscent of elemi oil, spearmint oil, citrus oils, etc. with a sweet, nutmeg-like undertone.

Mixes well with: fennel, tarragon, oregano, basil, marjoram, anise, parsley, angelica

ELEMI

Distilled from the gum-resin exudate of a tree found in the Philippines and South America, elemi has been used in Europe for 500 years in salves and liniments. It has many medicinal uses for healing wounds, the respiratory tract and inflammations. In perfumery it is a freshener and top note component.

Common name: Elemi

Family name: Burseraceae

Botanical name: Canarium Luzonicum

Dosha effect: V K–, P+

Taste: bitter, astringent, pungent

PD taste: pungent

Energy: heating, drying

Actions: expectorant, astringent, anti-inflammatory , vulnerary, stimulant

Tissues: respiratory, skin, nerves, muscles, lymph, joints

Indications: inflammation, wounds, congestion, bleeding

Warning: may cause skin irritation; use only small amount

Usage: massage oil, compress, salve, inhalation, liniments, perfume oil

Aroma: light, fresh, lemon-like, peppery odor which dries to a balsamic, green-woody and sweet-spicy afternote

Mixes well with: lemon, cajeput, basil, myrtle, eucalyptus, cinnamon, olibanum, labdanum, rosemary, lavender, sage

EUCALYPTUS

Light: Eucalyptus is one of the most commonly used essential oils. You could write a book on all its uses. There are over 700 varieties of eucalyptus, some growing to 500 feet, and they all possess similar properties. It is currently used in many allopathic medical preparations. It is one of the three best oils for use with any respiratory tract problem because the component eucalyptol is mucolytic (it relaxes the flow of mucous) and it excretes the eucalyptol out through the lung surface. Even if you take it internally in a tea form, eucalyptus will very quickly pass out of the body through the lungs, having its relaxing effect to the mucous membranes. As it is inhaled it gives an immediate effect; then again as it circulates out of the body. It is wonderful for acne because it reduces oil production and dries the tissue. It is thought to increase insulin production and help to balance the blood sugar.

As a child with asthma eucalyptus was part of my compress formula, including rosemary and camphor. I remember those smells and being wrapped in flannel so I could sleep through the night without gasping. The citriodora variety is thought to be best for children because of its lemony fresh smell. The globulous variety is stronger and more common. Often the heating effect of eucalyptus can be balanced by mixing it with a cooling oil such as lavender or peppermint (to reduce fever). It should be a part of everyone's medicine cabinet and first aid kit. Eucalyptus combines well with lemon for mental clarity, and with myrtle for building the immune system. Sometimes recommended in a compress over the spleen.

Common name: Eucalyptus

Family name: Myrtaceae

Botanical name: Eucalyptus Globulus, Citriodora, etc.

Dosha effect: K V–, P+

Taste: pungent

PD taste: pungent

Energy: heating/moisturizing

Actions: diaphoretic, decongestant, stimulant, antiseptic, antispasmodic, alterative, diuretic, expectorant, antipyretic, regenerative, lowers blood sugar, disinfects the air, increases concentration, deodorant, germicidal

Tissues: muscle, nerves, respiratory, blood, plasma

EUCALYPTUS (continued)

Indications: asthma, bronchitis, throat, sinus, kidney and bladder infections, fever, angina, rheumatism, neuritis, sore muscles, sluggishness, little intellectual enthusiasm, emotional overload, skin blemishes, acne, dandruff, tuberculosis, malaria, herpes simplex, skin ulcers, insect bites

Warning: do not take more than one or two drops a day internally

Usage: inhalation, aroma lamp, gargle, lozenge, massage oil, compress

Aroma: camphoraceous to lemony, medicinal smell

Mixes well with: rosemary, wintergreen, juniper, lavender, mint, cedarwood, citronella, geranium, tea tree, niaouli, angelica, elecampane

FENNEL

Fennel is another essential oil from the carrot family. Every lactating mother should have this oil at hand because it helps with milk production and eases colic. It is useful during pregnancy to prevent morning sickness, and is excellent for the traveler, helping to reduce or prevent sea sickness and jet lag. One of the most important carminative oils, it is useful for upset stomachs, gas, flatulence, indigestion and is traditionally used in Indian restaurants in herb form as an after dinner promoter of digestion. It has been recommended for reducing stomach acidity and prevention of ulcers. Fennel oil contains phyto-estrogens so its useful with PMS, menopause. Useful in toning the body because of its diuretic effect; it can be helpful in obesity. Often used in breast creams for tightening and enlarging.

Common name: Fennel

Family name: Umbelliferae

Botanical name: Foeniculum Vulgare or Valgra Dulce

Other name: Shatapushpa

Dosha effect: V P K=

Taste: sweet, pungent

PD taste: sweet

Energy: cooling (slightly), moisturizing

Actions: carminative, diuretic, anti-spasmodic, stimulant, female tonic

Tissues: plasma, blood, muscles, marrow, endocrine, GI tract

Indications: indigestion, low agni, abdominal pain, cramps or gas, difficult or burning urination, children's colic, cold symptoms, abcesses, PMS, weak, irregular periods, stress, nervousness, overindulgence in alcohol and nicotine, hangover

Warning: none

Usage: food, massage oil, bath, aroma lamp, inhalations, tea

Aroma: (sweet, only cultivated) very sweet, but slightly earthy or peppery-spicy odor and a clean, sweet aromatic dryout, a hint of fruity-fresh topnote in fresh oils

Mixes well with: anise, caraway, lavender, chamomiles, angelica, cardamon, clove, orange, ginger

FIR

Fir is used by many massage therapists because it is a relaxant to the nervous system and to muscle spasm. It can be a great substitute for pine, and milder on the skin. It is a favorite to spritz the house around Christmas time because of its refreshing smell, reminding us of the deep forest. The oil is antiseptic, very good for the respiratory tract. Because of its fresh, clean, outdoorsy smell it is a wonderful addition to aftershave lotion.

Common name: Fir

Family name: Coniferae (Pine)

Botanical name: Abies Balsamea

Dosha effect: K V–, P+, (V+ in excess)

Taste: pungent, bitter

PD taste: pungent

Energy: heating, drying

Actions: antiseptic, expectorant

Tissues: muscular

Indications: back pain, joint pain, tissue congestion.

Warning: can cause irritation in people with sensitive skin

Usage: massage oil, aftershave, perfume, cologne

Aroma: refreshingly balsamic, slightly fatty or oily with a powerful pine forest odor, a peculiar fruity-balsamic undertone

Mixes well with: birch, juniper, wintergreen, lavender, pine, cedarwood, musk, citrus, labdanum, patchouli

FRANKINCENSE

Sometimes called olibanum, frankincense is one of the first spices brought back from the East. It is gathered from the trunk and stems of small trees which grow in the Arabian peninsula, India, and northern Africa. One of the original gifts to the Christ Child, frankincense preserves spiritual energy, is an enhancement for meditation, and can help to maintain a clear mind. It is still used ritually in the Catholic church during religious ceremonies for devotional cleansing and purification of the soul. It was an important ingredient in the preservation of the bodies of the pharaohs. It is still used in cosmetics today because of its regulating effect on mature skin. An important oil for anointing the dead and dying, for assisting in transition and keeping the soul connected to its divine essence. It is excellent for the sixth chakra, assisting in altering perception of truth and promoting clairvoyance. Because it provides mental stability, it is used to ease depression, often combined with bergamot and geranium.

Common name: Frankincense

Family name: Burseraceae

Botanical name: Boswellia Thurifera

Other name: Olibanum

Dosha effect: K V–, P+

Taste: bitter, pungent, astringent, sweet

PD taste: pungent

Energy: heating, drying

Actions: alterative, analgesic, rejuvenative, anti-inflammatory, disinfectant, antiseptic, astringent

Tissues: muscle, fat

Indications: wounds, bronchitis, colds, sinusitis, wrinkles

Warning: always dilute

Usage: bath, lotion, patches

Aroma: strongly diffusive, fresh terpene, almost green, lemon-like, reminiscent of green unripe apple peels, certain peppery-ness is mellowed with a rich, sweet-woody, balsamic undertone.

Mixes well with: myrrh, rose, sandalwood, dhavana, champa, citrus, violet, cinnamon, musk, labdanum, neroli, vetiver

GARLIC AND ONION

Both oils are highly rejuvenative, especially for the nerve tissue. They combine well, as in cooking; however no one in their right mind would ever use this oil for aromatherapy, although it is used extensively in medicine and in the food flavoring industry. It is available at reasonable price. At one time we thought it would be wonderful to sell every oil that was on the market, and even included these two oils in our **Earth Essentials** price list. While we were carrying the oils to a trade show in Anaheim, one of them leaked in the trunk of the car, and in spite of our efforts to deodorize, the car was almost unusable. We almost lost a friendship over that oil. Subsequently, we declined to carry it with us or in our line. We now feel that the fresh plants contain sufficient qualities of the oils to provide most Americans abundant garlic and onion oil simply though their eating habits.

Common name: Garlic
Botanical name: Allium Sativum
Common name: Onion
Botanical name: Allium Cepa
Family name: Liliacae
Dosha effect: K V–, Pitta+
Taste: pungent and sweet
PD taste: pungent
Energy: heating and drying
Actions: stimulant, carminative, expectorant, alterative, antispasmodic, aphrodisiac, disinfectant, rejuvenative
Tissues: all tissues, systems—digestive, respiratory, nervous, reproductive, circulatory
Indications: colds, skin disease, parasites, joint problems, fluid retention
Warning: odor nearly impossible to counteract; not recommended
Usage: cooking, cough medicine, food
Aroma: obnoxiously sulfuraceous with the distinct intense smell of the crushed plant bulb
Mixes well with: ginger, black pepper, cumin, coriander, eucalyptus, food

GERANIUM

Geranium is another oil that is a special gift for women because of its effect on the menstrual cycle. It is balancing, calming, and anti-depressive. An important essential oil during menopause, due to its phyto-estrogen components; it is used in skin care for maintaining youthful beautiful skin. Very helpful in any dehydrating skin condition like eczema. Its good for almost all skin problems because of its balancing effect. Our 17-year-old son enjoys using this oil mixed with sandalwood and rosewood in equal amounts. He maintains that it helps to keep him centered, calm, and puts people at ease.

Common name: Geranium

Family name: Geraniaceae

Botanical name: Pelargonium Ordorantissium
Roseum Graveolens

Other Name: Rose Geranium

Dosha effect: P K–, V

Taste: sweet, astringent

PD taste: sweet

Energy: cooling, moisturizing

Actions: antidepressant, nervine,
aphrodisiac, menopause
hormone balancer, antiseptic,
anti-inflammatory, insect repellent

Tissues: nerve, muscle, reproductive, skin

Indications: wounds, menopause, eczemas, shingles, tongue infections, stomatitis, facial neuralgia, irritated skin, acne, PMS

Warning: none

Usage: lotion, inhalation, compress, perfumes, massage oil, bath, aromatherapy

Aroma: intensely earthy-herbaceous, somewhat sharp-rosy, foliage-green odor of great tenacity

Mixes well with: rose, clary sage, rosewood, sandalwood, lavender, champa, musk, vanilla, bergamot, patchouli, clove

GINGER

Ginger is one of the most commonly used herbs in Ayurveda and Chinese medicine. Because of its digestive properties, it is without peer in cases of illness due to poor absorption and assimilation. Being a root, it is very grounding and centering; it's also warming. Just the simple addition of moderate quantities of ginger can increase metabolism. It's wonderful for regulating the blood, for motion sickness, weight loss; it is helpful in bringing any condition into balance. For sea sickness, air sickness or problems in balance use it on a small circular bandage behind the ear. Light often adds it to her bath on cold mornings and to daily skin massage lotion in the winter.

Common name: Ginger

Family name: Zingiberaceae (Ginger)

Botanical name: Zingiber Officinalis

Dosha effect: V K–, P+

Taste: pungent, sweet

PD taste: sweet

Energy: warming/drying

Actions: stimulant, diaphoretic, antidepressant, expectorant, antiemetic, analgesic, carminative

Tissues: all tissue elements

Indications: colds, flus, indigestion, vomiting, belching, abdominal pain, laryngitis, arthritis, hemorrhoids, headaches, impotence, diarrhea, heart disease, poor memory

Warning: don't use if inflammatory skin diseases, high fever, bleeding, or ulcers are present

Usage: tea, cooking, massage, compress

Aroma: warm, but fresh, woody, spicy, with a peculiar resemblance to orange, lemon, lemongrass, coriander weed oil in the initial, fresh topnotes; the undertone is sweet, heavy, rich, tenacious, almost balsamic floral

Mixes well with: black pepper, eucalyptus, juniper, cypress, rose, cedarwood, coriander, all citrus, neroli

GRAPEFRUIT

Light: I am normally not attracted to the citrus oils because their top notes go directly to my head, making me spacey, but this oil is excellent for stimulating self esteem, creating euphoria, and self-worth. In skin care it can be used for herpes, acne, edema, cellulite. It mixes well with lemon and bergamot for a morning uplifting bath. The seed oil is quite expensive and is an expressed oil. It is being used for candidiasis, bacterial infection and parasites, as well as in cosmetics. Oil of grapefruit can be very helpful with digestive problems and may be a stimulant to the gall bladder and the production of bile in the liver.

Common name: Grapefruit
Family name: Rutacea (Rue)
Botanical name: Citrus Pardisi - Deucumana
Dosha effect: K V–, P+
Taste: Sweet, sour
PD taste: sour
Energy: warming/drying
Actions: stimulant, carminative, diuretic, regulates eating disorders
Tissues: muscle, lymphatic, digestive, nerve, hepatic
Indications: digestive problems, lymphatic system, secretions, obesity, water retention, liver and gall bladder, cellulite, depressing mornings, self-doubt
Warning: phototoxic - exposure to sun may blemish skin
Usage: cooking, perfumes, lotion, massage oil, drinks, deserts, inhalation, diffuser
Aroma: fresh - citrusy, rather sweet odor like the fruit rind
Mixes well with: all citrus and lavender

HYSSOP

Hyssop is mentioned in the Bible many times and is one of the oldest herbs used by man. It is used for colds, sinus and respiratory problems, and is a balancer and regulator of high blood pressure. It has expectorant qualities and can be helpful in heavy catarrhal conditions. It is a carminative herb and is an ingredient of Chartreuse liquor.

Common name: Hyssop

Family name: Labiatae

Botanical name: Hyssopus Officinalis

Dosha effect: K–, P+

Taste: pungent, bitter

PD taste: pungent

Energy: heating, drying

Actions: diaphoretic, diuretic, carminative, anthelmintic, vulnerary, alterative, mental stimulant, centering, stomachic, antiseptic

Tissues: digestive, skin, respiratory, kidney

Indications: lung ailments (chronic catarrh), congestion, fevers, poor circulation and digestion, external wounds, high/low blood pressure, confusion

Warning: do not use in cases of epilepsy or pregnancy

Usage: compress, inhalation, bath, skin lotion, food and drink

Aroma: a powerful, somewhat sharp but sweet-camphoraceous odor, with warm-aromatic, spicy undertone

Mixes well with: eucalyptus, myrtle, lavender, citrus, rosemary, sage, camphor, juniper, cajeput, laurel (bay), clary sage, geranium

JASMINE

Jasmine is one of the most expensive oils. Most readily available as an absolute, it is sometimes found in CO_2 form. It is especially calming for those times when you are feeling disconnected, out of control, not knowing what to do. The smell of this oil can bring us balance, possibilities, hope, connectedness, confidence. It is very balancing to both male and female hormones. Very attracting to the opposite sex. An excellent aphrodisiac. May prevent uterine problems; helpful in skin care. Excellent brain stimulant.

Common name: Jasmine

Family name: Oleacea (Olive family)

Botanical name: Jasmimum Grandiflorum

Other name: Jati

Dosha effect: P K–, V+

Taste: bitter, sweet

PD taste: pungent

Energy: cooling, moisturizing

Actions: alternative, refrigerant, emmenagogue, nervine, antibacterial, aphrodisiac, antidepressant

Tissues: plasma, blood, bone, marrow, reproductive

Indications: emotional disturbance, headache, fever, sunstroke, conjunctivitis, childbirth, dermatitis, burning urethra, bleeding disorders, bacterial or viral infections, cancer of lymph nodes, bone cancer, dry skin, dermatitis, anxiety, lack of confidence

Warning: do not take internally, has been extracted

Usage: perfume, lotion, aroma lamp, bath, massage

Aroma: generally warm, intensely floral, somewhat indolic-sharp, but immensely rich and tenacious, herbaceous-sweet, fatty green, tea-like undertones

Mixes well with: rose, sandalwood, all citrus, juniper, cypress, champa, chamomile, ylang ylang, cinnamon, rosewood, violet

JUNIPERBERRY

Light: There have been periods in my life when this oil has been a savior. I use it quite frequently in my morning bath, combined with orange cypress, because of its strong diuretic property. Because of its heating qualities and the movement of fluid, it is wonderful for both Vata and Kapha arthritis and rheumatism. Juniper can be an aid in promoting menstruation and useful in bladder infections.

Common name:	Juniperberry
Family name:	Cupressacea
Botanical name:	Juniperus Communis
Other name:	Hapusha
Dosha effect:	K V–, P+, (V+ in excess)
Taste:	pungent, bitter, sweet
PD taste:	pungent
Energy:	heating
Actions:	diuretic, diaphoretic, carminative, analgesic, stimulant, disinfectant, astringent, bactericidal
Tissues:	plasma, blood, muscle, fat, bone, marrow, nerves, lymph, uterus
Indications:	dropsy, edema, sciatica, lumbago, arthritis, rheumatism, swollen joints, diabetes, weak digestion, weak immune system, dysmenorrhea
Warning:	not to be used for acute kidney infections or during pregnancy
Usage:	bath, lotion, aroma lamp, weight loss formulas, massage oil, lotion, inhalation
Aroma:	fresh, yet warm, rich-balsamic, woody-sweet and pine-needle-like odor
Mixes well with:	all citrus, cypress, eucalyptus, cajaput, labdanum, opoponox, elemi, clary sage, lavender, benzoin

LAVENDER

Author Susanne Fischer-Rizzi says that lavender has 167 medicinal uses which have been tested. It falls very central to the chemical properties chart and so is good for almost any imbalance. It is definitely the most important oil to have in a travel kit or first aid package. If you are tired and stressed out, it will relax you. If you are depressed, it will uplift you. If you are angry and hypertensive, it will calm you. It is one of the essential oils that is excellent for children. It is wonderful for blending because you can use as it a modifier, middle note, or to cover any unpleasant oil whose therapeutic effect you want to equalize in a blend. Because of its antipyretic and diaphoretic properties, it is excellent for fever. Our son developed a fever while we were traveling somewhere in New Mexico, and Light pulled over and massaged him with a combination of blue chamomile and lavender (quite a strong mixture—it may have been as much as 30% essential oil to 70% vegetable oil), and his fever of 105 went down to normal in just one hour. He was able to sleep the night and was feeling pretty good the next day.

Common name: Lavender, French

Family name: Labiatae (Mint Family)

Botanical name: Lavendula Officinalis

Other name: Angustifolia

Dosha effect: P K–, V o

Taste: pungent

PD taste: pungent

Energy: slightly cooling/neutral

Actions: carminative, diuretic, antispasmodic, antiseptic, analgesic, galactogogue, stimulant, balancing, diuretic

Tissues: all elements

Indications: burns, wounds, insect bites, eczemas, dermatitis, boils, leg ulcers, fever blisters, herpes, rheumatism, neuritis, lumbago, ear infections, headache, yeast infection, athlete's foot, colds, flu, bronchitis, motion sickness, gall bladder disorders, high blood pressure, nervous heart, stress, insomnia, irritability, mood swings, dry skin, acne, fluid retention, hair loss, dandruff

Warning: do not use with preparations containing iodine or iron

Usage: all: aroma lamp, inhalation, bath, lotion, massage oil, sprayer, food, laundry scent, pillow; can be used directly on the skin

LAVENDER (continued)

Aroma: rich, sweet-herbaceous, floral odor, woody-herby undertones and coumarin-like sweetness

Mixes well with: all oils, but especially citrus, geranium, rose, neroli, clove, patchouli, rosemary, clary sage and conifers; useful blended with any unpleasant or strong-smelling oil

LEMON BALM

Lemon balm (also known as melissa) is one of the rarest, least available, and often most misrepresented of essential oils. Because it takes as much as 12,000 pounds of lemon balm to make one pound of balm oil, its cost can be comparable to rose. If you are paying less, you are probably purchasing an adulterated product with some balm oil and a large quantity of citronella as an additive. The real thing is one of the most important oils for the immune system, allergies, stimulation of the thymus, and lymphatic drainage. Its components are especially effective with virus and various forms of herpes, and good for the digestion, especially the liver and gallbladder. Is also a regulator of the hormonal system. It is excellent for couch potatoes who do not know what to do with their lives, and can be an effective inhalation when you are working on your purpose or setting goals. Helpful with all stagnated tissue, bruises, obesity and an especially good hair oil for dandruff.

Common name: Lemon Balm

Family name: Labiatae

Botanical name: Melissa Officinalis

Other name: Melissa

Dosha effect: K P–, V o

Taste: pungent, sour-sweet

PD taste: pungent

Energy: cooling/moisturizing

Actions: diaphoretic, carminative, nervine, antispasmodic, sedative, antipyretic

Tissues: nerve, blood, lymphatic muscle, organ tissue, spleen

Indications: infant and child afflictions, fever, colds, flus, melancholy, menopause

Warning: beware adulterations

Usage: shampoo, perfumes, lotion, massage oils, shower gel, compress, aroma lamp

Aroma: citral-like, fresh topnote with a sweet herbaceous odor

Mixes well with: geranium, champa, eucalyptus, lavender, basil, bergamot, rosewood

LEMON OIL

Lemon is one of the most common oils and is most often cold pressed because of its availability. It has a fresh, clean, familiar smell. It is a favorite additive to detergents, dish soap, household cleansers, bleach, and is a wonderful addition to foods. Some countries require that the lemon oil offered in their pharmacies contain a certain percentage of natural citrol which can vary due to weather and harvesting conditions. Occasionally, batches are adulterated with chemically-produced citrol to meet this requirement. A more common practice is the intentional removal of terpenes which produces an oil which is much gentler and more suitable for skin care use. These oils will be labeled "terpene free." More rare, and expensive, is steam-distilled lemon oil which has an indefinite shelf life (as opposed to one to two years) and is also the most suitable for skin care.

Lemon oil is excellent for concentration. Its clean, refreshing energy is a stimulant to the nervous system. In blending, it can be very helpful to add life to a mixture which is flat. It is a stimulant to the immune system and a blood cleanser; especially useful for viruses. I've seen it combined with niaouli and administered internally for treatment of earache; it was successful when no other oil combination, internal or external, seemed to have effect.

Common name:	Lemon
Family name:	Rutacea
Botanical name:	Citrus Limonum
Dosha effect:	P V–, K o
Taste:	sour, sweet
PD taste:	sour
Energy:	cooling/drying
Actions:	expectorant, carminative, astringent, stimulant, antiseptic, deputative, antivirus, antidepressant
Tissues:	skin, nerves
Indications:	oily skin, digestive problems, infectious diseases, viral diseases, leucocyte formation, anemia, hypertension, hyperviscosity, low immunity, cellulitis, anxiety, lymph, gall bladder or liver congestion
Warning:	may cause irritation to sensitive skin; possible phototoxin
Usage:	all, especially: food (desserts), bath, aromatherapy, lotion, shampoo, conditioner, inhalation, massage oil

LEMON OIL (continued)

Aroma: very light, fresh and sweet odor of short duration, reminiscent of the ripe peel

Mixes well with: all citrus, juniper, cypress, lavender, labdanum, dhavana, jatamansi, mints, elemi, petitgrain, neroli

LEMONGRASS

Bryan: Lemongrass is very high in water-soluble vitamin A, and is excellent for the immune system, the lymphatics, the blood and circulation. It is an excellent antidepressant, and it works wonders with connective tissues and back pain. Known to assist with headache relief, kidney infections and swelling, the oil can also be used for stimulating the thyroid. Lemongrass is very prolific (grows up to six feet high), harvests six months after planting, and can be cut three to four times a year. I bought four plants from a nursery and at the end of one year those plants had increased to 84. I separated them and transplanted them again and nine months later I now have over 300 plants forming a hedge around my pool patio. Four million pounds are distilled worldwide each year. It is used extensively by the cosmetics industry for soaps and skin care products. It's one of the oils least tolerated by insects and is great in any mosquito repellent spray or added to your pet's shampoo.

Common name:	Lemongrass
Family name:	Graminae
Botanical name:	Cymbopogon Citratus
Dosha effect:	P K–, V o
Taste:	pungent, bitter
PD taste:	pungent
Energy:	cooling/moisturizing
Actions:	diuretic, diaphoretic, refrigerant, antiseptic, stimulant, tonic, astringent
Tissues:	blood, muscle, marrow, lymphatic
Indications:	weak digestion, flatulence, intestinal infections, bladder and kidney infections, fluid retention, edema, varicose veins, oily skin, large pores, poor concentration, long trips, difficult mornings
Warning:	may irritate sensitive skin when used as compress or facial oil
Usage:	compress, cooking, massage oil, aroma lamp, bath, shampoo, inhalation
Aroma:	very strong, fresh grassy lemon-type herbaceous or tea-like odor
Mixes well with:	bergamot, rosemary, lavender, juniper, hyssop, pine, rosewood

LIME

Lime can be used externally as a disinfectant for cuts or infections in a 15% solution (15% essential oil and 85% water or oil), or internally to fight viruses. In body care it has a deodorizing effect and it tightens skin and connective tissue. Known to have carminative and diuretic qualities, lime may be used as a food flavoring and in men's toiletries.

Common name: Lime

Family name: Rutacea

Botanical name: Citrus Aurantifolia

Dosha effect: P K–, V+

Taste: sour, bitter

PD taste: sour

Energy: cooling/drying

Actions: refrigerant, carminative, expectorant, stimulant, diuretic, antiseptic, antispasmodic, antidepressant, tonic, virus protection

Tissues: skin, digestive, respiratory, nervous system

Indications: hot climates, poor digestion, lymph congestion, gall bladder congestion, liver problems, anemia, obesity, asthma, bronchitis, anxiety, depression, infections

Warning: do not use on skin when sunbathing

Usage: aroma lamp, massage oil, bath, conditioner, inhalation, food, aftershave

Aroma: intensely fresh, rich and sweet, peel-like

Mixes well with: all citrus, lavender, lemongrass, petitgrain, rosewood

MANDARIN

Mandarin is a variety of tangerine. It is very calming and soothing for stress. It can be combined with orange to make a "happy oil" to bring cheer into the atmosphere. It is good for children and is a nice addition to massage oil for people who need a familiar smell. The aroma is excellent for digestion. It can be used on the skin for teenagers who are growing quickly and developing stretch marks, and for stretch marks during pregnancy.

Common name: Mandarin Red

Family name: Rutacea (Rue family)

Botanical name: Citrus Reticulata

Dosha effect: P K–, V+ (in excess)

Taste: sweet, sour, bitter

PD taste: sour

Energy: cooling/drying

Actions: calming, antispasmodic, nervine, astringent, hypnotic

Tissues: nerves, skin, digestive

Indications: nervous tension, insomnia, epilepsy

Warning: all citrus must be used with care when in direct sunlight

Usage: massage oil, compress, lotion, aroma lamp, cooking

Aroma: intensely sweet, not very fresh odor, sometimes amine-like, "fishy" topnote, rich, neroli-like, floral undertone

Mixes well with: jasmine, neroli, dhavana, cypress, frankincense, geranium, rosewood, petitgrain

MARJORAM

Most popular these days as an anti-aphrodisiac; used extensively and defensively by those women wishing a decrease in advances by their spouses. It also works well with tension and letting go. Not the most pleasant of smells, it can be masked with lighter flowery scents such as lavender, champa and citrus, when making a blend for migraines and muscle pain. It can be useful for sinus congestion, indigestion, gas. A dilator of blood vessels, it can stimulate menstruation and should not be taken during pregnancy. Light made the unfortunate mistake of using marjoram oil to clean our motor home refrigerator, and for six months afterwards all of our food smelled like marjoram. Our son would audibly groan if anyone opened the refrigerator door for food. It was a great inducement to eat in restaurants while we were traveling.

Common name: Marjoram

Family name: Labiatae (Mint family)

Botanical name: Origanum Majorana

Dosha effect: K V–, P+

Taste: pungent, bitter

PD taste: pungent

Energy: heating

Actions: stimulant, antispasmodic diaphoretic, emmenagogue, hypotensor, vasodilator, analgesic, sedative, anti-aphrodisiac

Tissues: nerve, skin, reproductive, circulatory

Indications: emotional exhaustion, migraine with neck tension, excessive sexual drive, sore muscles, congestion, poor digestion, flatulence, intestinal cramps, high blood pressure, PMS, insomnia

Warning: marjoram will cut down sexual desire; too much will cause lethargy

Usage: massage oil, lotion, bath, compress, coolant, inhalant

Aroma: warm-spicy aromatic-camphoraceous and woody odor, reminiscent of nutmeg and cardamon

Mixes well with: anything which will mask its smell

MYRRH

Myrrh is one of the oldest of essential oils. The oil is made from the gum resin of a bush that grows in Arabia and Africa. One of the gifts brought to the Christ Child by the Magi, it is used to preserve divine essence, and to maintain and support that state of grace. The oil is excellent for Kapha emotions, and for people who are afraid to speak up about their feelings. The oil creates confidence and awareness. Because it moves fluids, it is excellent for weight loss. Used originally to preserve the bodies of the pharaohs, it continues to be a preservative and restorer of youth and is used extensively in cosmetics for mature skin and the prevention of wrinkles. Myrrh has very strong antiseptic and antifungal qualities. Its centering properties make it an excellent inhalation for compulsive eaters, in part because it connects them with real issues and does not allow them to hide behind their food.

Common name: Myrrh

Family name: Burseracea (Resin)

Botanical name: Commophora Myrrha

Other name: Bola (Indian)

Dosha effect: K V–, P+

Taste: bitter, pungent

PD Taste: pungent

Energy: heating

Actions: alterative, analgesic, emmenagogue, rejuvenative, astringent, expectorant, antispasmodic, antiseptic

Tissues: all tissues

Indications: amenorrhea, dysmenorrhea, menopause, cough, asthma, bronchitis, arthritis, rheumatism, traumatic injuries, ulcerated surfaces, anemia, pyorrhea

Warning: aggravates Pitta (excess heat in the body)

Usage: lotion, salve, massage oil, weight reduction formulas

Aroma: warm-spicy, showing a very peculiar sharp-balsamic, slightly medicinal topnote; the sweetness increases to a deep, warm-spicy and aromatic dryout, which is unique

Mixes well with: frankincense, orange, tangerine, juniper, cypress, geranium, musk, pine, patchouli and heavy flower oils

MYRTLE

Myrtle is produced from an evergreen bush that grows around the Mediterranean. It is often helpful with allergies, because it adjusts the mind into tolerance of the psychological component (someone or something the person is irritated with). Its clarifying effects can help us gain insight. It can be very helpful in meditation. It is also useful with addictions and other dependency problems. Myrtle is always part of Light's formula for stopping smoking, drug abuse, or repetitive emotional cycles. Used in skin care as a cleanser and toner, it is especially effective with Pitta skin.

Common name: Myrtle

Family name: Myrtaceae

Botanical name: Myrtus Communis

Dosha effect: K P–, V+

Taste: sweet, pungent

PD taste: pungent

Energy: warming, drying

Actions: expectorant, antiseptic, astringent, tonic, strengthens meditation, balancing

Tissues: respiratory

Indications: colds, bronchitis, coughs, tuberculosis, smoker's cough, sinus infection, urinary infections, respiratory tract ailments, addictions, transitions, oily skin, acne

Warning: none

Usage: compress, massage oil, salve, diffusor, humidifier, cooking, inhalations

Aroma: strongly camphoraceous-spicy, also sweet-herbaceous and fresh body notes

Mixes well with: jatamansi, jasmine, sandalwood, lemon, dhavana, keawa, rose, eucalyptus, camphor, clove bud, cinnamon, bergamot, lavender, rosemary, clary sage, hyssop, lime, bay

NEROLI

Neroli is made from the flowers of the orange tree, and is named after a famous Italian princess who wore it as her signature perfume. Sometimes steam distilled, often sold as an absolute or more costly CO_2 derivative, it is one of the most expensive of oils. It is also one of the most intense-smelling oils, best appreciated in very mild dilutions. Neroli connects you to the God self within. It gives confidence and strength to the mind, has relaxing properties which help with sleeplessness, and can be an ally during times of stress. It has a special affinity for the female immune system, and is part of all our female immune regulatory formulas. It helps women in almost any stage of transition, reduces cramps, assists in menopause, is excellent with depression, anger, the heart. In skin care, neroli is anti-Pitta, helping with inflammation and broken vessels.

Common name: Neroli
Family name: Rutacea
Botanical name: Citrus Bigaradia or Awrantium
Other name: Orange Blossom
Dosha effect: P V–, K+
Taste: sweet, bitter
PD taste: sweet
Energy: cooling/moisturizing
Actions: antispasmodic, antiseptic, calmative, carminative, tonic, stimulant, antidepressant, germicidal
Tissues: skin, nerve, reproductive, circulatory
Indications: headaches, flatulence, tachycardia, nervous heart, PMS, emotional instability, insomnia, test anxiety, hopelessness, aging skin, dermatitis
Warning: avoid internal use of absolute
Usage: perfume, bath, lotion, massage oil, inhalation, aroma lamp
Aroma: very powerful, light and refreshing, floral with a peculiar sweet-terpeney topnote but poor tenacity; top note material extraordinaire
Mixes well with: rose, lavender, sandalwood, jasmine, cypress, juniper and all citrus, rosewood, petitgrain, chamomile, everlasting, cardamon, myrrh, opoponox

NIAOULI

Niaouli is a member of the melaleuca family, all of which are known for their abilities against infections: bacterial, fungal, yeast and virus. Lemon in combination with Niaouli can be an internal remedy for ear infection. It is excellent for the respiratory system and urinary tract, like eucalyptus and tea tree oil, and it works well as a liniment for various types of arthritic pains. Niaouli is often used in aphrodisiac blends. It is a stimulant and tonic for digestion and circulation, and has analgesic properties similar to clove. Some sources report that it can influence and stimulate vivid dream activity. Too much of this oil can decrease your brain activity because of its grounding properties. Use with care, no more than one to two drops a day.

Common name: Niaouli

Family name: Myrtaceae (Myrtle)

Botanical name: Melaleuca Virisiflora

Dosha effect: P K–, V+

Taste: bitter, astringent, sweet

PD taste: sweet

Energy: cooling, moisturizing

Actions: balancing, antiseptic, stimulant, expectorant

Tissues: nerve, skin, respiratory

Indications: bronchial problems, urinary tract problems, colds, flus, bronchitis, coughs, wounds, ear infections, rheumatism, acne, burns, earache

Warning: do not use directly on skin; always dilute

Usage: lotion, massage oils, aroma lamp, salve, inhalations

Aroma: strong, fresh, sweet-camphoraceous but cooling odor, reminiscent of eucalyptus and cardamon, however, less spicy

Mixes well with: lemon, tea tree, myrtle, hyssop, eucalyptus, rosemary, St. Johns wort, and orange

NUTMEG

Nutmeg oil is steam distilled from the dried fruits. In small quantities it can stimulate brain activity, digestion, blood flow, nerve impulses. Beware of excess use as it can cause dulling of the brain. Useful for grounding, it can calm and strengthen when added to a blend. It has long been a favorite in men's aftershaves, soaps and perfumes.

Common name: Nutmeg

Family name: Myrtaceae

Botanical name: Myristica Fragrans

Other name: Jatiphala

Dosha effect: V K–, P+

Taste: pungent

PD taste: pungent

Energy: heating

Actions: astringent, carminative, sedative, nervine, aphrodisiac, stimulant, helps dream recall

Tissues: plasma, muscle, marrow, and nerve, reproductive

Indications: poor absorption, abdominal pain and distention, diarrhea, dysentery, intestinal gas, insomnia, nervous disorders, impotence, poor circulation, menstrual irregularity, rheumatism, low energy

Warning: avoid during pregnancy, high Pitta; toxic in large quantities, *as little as one teaspoon may be fatal*

Usage: lotions, toothache, aphrodisiac, massage oil, aroma lamp

Aroma: light, fresh, warm-spicy and aromatic odor, a distinctly terpeney topnote and a rich, sweet-spicy, warm bodynote; undertone and dryout is somewhat woody

Mixes well with: bay, lavender, cumin, Peru balsam, cinnamon

ORANGE

Orange is one of the least expensive oils produced, pressed from the skin of the orange fruit which is abundantly available. It has similar properties to neroli, although it is not as fine. It has a very familiar scent because of its abundant industrial and food flavor use. It is particularly useful for skin care, especially for cellulite (which is sometimes called orange skin because of the dimpling that resembles the skin of an orange). It is very good for dry skin conditions and calluses. It is wonderful for opening the heart, is beneficial for sadness, nervousness and anxiety. Depending on the person it can be relaxing or energizing.

Common name: Orange

Family name: Rutacea (Rue)

Botanical name: Citrus Aurantium

Dosha effect: V K–, P+

Taste: pungent, bitter

PD taste: pungent

Energy: heating

Actions: carminative, expectorant, stimulant, anti-inflammatory, heart tonic, disinfectant, antipyretic

Tissues: all tissues

Indications: weak digestion, gallbladder blockage, heart muscle spasm, irregular heartbeat, bladder and kidney disorders, fever, gingivitis, cellulite, dry skin, aging skin, anxiety, sadness, self-consciousness

Warning: may irritate sensitive skin when exposed to sun

Usage: bath, massage oil, aroma lamp, perfumes, spritzer, cooking

Aroma: sweet, light and fresh, fruity-aldehydic odor and flavor, distinctly reminiscent of the odor from a scratched sweet orange peel

Mixes well with: coriander, ylang ylang, sandalwood, juniper, cypress and neroli, lavender, rosemary, clary sage, oakmoss, labdanum, frankincense

PALMAROSA

Light: Palmarosa is used widely in Ayurvedic skin care. It is good for all skin types because it is a cellular stimulator and supports all cell regulation. It's highly antiseptic, calming, uplifting, and antidepressive. It can be a stimulant to the endocrine system and to lymphatic drainage. Some people love the odor, but I find it quite sedating. I prefer it when it's fresh, because after one year it becomes quite strong. To use it then I must mix it with other sweet oils.

Common name: Palmarosa

Family name: Graminae (Grass)

Botanical name: Cymbocodan Martin

Dosha effect: V P K–

Taste: astringent, bitter sweet

PD taste: sweet

Energy: cooling, moisturizing

Actions: antiseptic, cell regenerator, stimulant, moisturizer, aphrodisiac

Tissues: skin, nerves, digestive, endocrine, lymph

Indications: acne, dermatitis, general skin care, dry skin, digestive problems, wrinkles

Warning: none

Usage: bath drops, inhalation, facial lotion, massage oil, ointments

Aroma: sweet, floral-rosy, various undertones or topnotes according to quality and age of oil

Mixes well with: rose, geranium, frankincense, jasmine, myrrh, lemon, champa, jatamansi, chamomiles, rosewood, oakmoss, all citrus

PARSLEY SEED OIL

This oil is used commonly by the food industry in soups and sauces. It is excellent to counter bad breath, especially after a meal of strong garlic dishes. The oil is a strong diuretic without causing dehydration. The oil can be made from the plant or the seed, the seed being more costly. Parsley is excellent for the circulation and is known to eliminate broken capillaries in combination with rose oil and cold compresses. An oil made from the leaves retains the fresh herb smell and is used exclusively in food flavoring.

Common name: Parsley

Family name: Umbelliferae (Carrot)

Botanical name: Petroselinum Sativum

Dosha effect: K V–, P+

Taste: pungent, bitter

PD taste: pungent

Energy: heating/drying

Actions: diuretic, emmenagogue, carminative, lithotriptic, laxative, antispasmodic

Tissues: plasma, blood, muscles

Indications: dropsy, edema, swollen glands, swollen breasts, amenorrhea, dysmenorrhea, gall stones, kidney stones, lumbago, sciatica

Warning: avoid if acute inflammation of kidneys or female reproductive system, or if high Pitta condition is present

Usage: compress, cooking, massage, bath

Aroma: seed: warm-woody, spicy, somewhat herbaceous but not at all reminiscent of the parsley herb

Mixes well with: juniper, cajeput, rosemary, neroli, rose, dill, myrtle, tea tree, oakmoss, clary sage

PATCHOULI

Patchouli is the oil most associated with the sixties, often used by people to cover the smell of whatever they were smoking. It's extremely useful for skin infections. It has traditional use as a moth repellent. Patchouli is often added to perfumes because of its aphrodisiac affect. Its thickness makes it a natural fixative, and it seems to be particularly effective with fungal, yeast and bacterial infections. It can also be useful as a mouthwash or a gargle.

Common name: Patchouli

Family name: Labiatae (Mint)

Botanical name: Pogostemom Cablim

Dosha effect: V P–, K+

Taste: sweet, bitter

PD taste: sweet

Energy: warming

Actions: regenerative, fungicidal, decongestant, antidepressant, aphrodisiac, antiseptic, tonic

Tissues: skin

Indications: acne, dermatitis, eczema, aged skin, cracked and chapped skin, impetigo, seborrhea, dandruff, neurasthenia, anxiety, yeast infections of mouth and vagina, viral infection, wounds

Warning: beware of imitation fragrance oils

Usage: mixed with tea tree oil as a mouthwash for infection; as a douche solution for vaginal infections, massage oil, salves, baths, and moth repellent

Aroma: extremely rich, sweet herbaceous, aromatic-spicy and woody-balsamic; almost wine-like, ethereal-floral sweetness in initial notes, bodynotes display outstanding richness, a root-like note with a delicate earthiness, the sweeter fragrances bring a balance to its earthy base note

Mixes well with: ylang ylang, lemon, musk, neroli and rose

PENNYROYAL

A member of the mint family, pennyroyal has a very spicy, aromatic top note, which makes some people nauseous. There have been several deaths from use of this oil as an aborti-factant, and so it has a bad reputation in aromatherapy. *It is not recommended for internal use and is definitely contra-indicated in pregnancy.* Best used externally as spritzer or lotion for insects. Pennyroyal seems to keep ticks and fleas away from dogs.

Common name: Pennyroyal

Botanical name: Mentha Pelegium

Dosha effect: V K–, P+

Taste: pungent

PD taste: pungent

Energy: heating/drying

Actions: insect repellent, antivenomous

Tissues: none

Indications: hysteria, nervousness, headaches, fleas, mosquitos

Warning: avoid use during pregnancy; best not used internally

Usage: insect repellent, spritzer

Aroma: very fresh, strong, herbaceous-minty but not very bitter odor

Mixes well with: rosemary, pine, lavender, citrus, lemongrass, citronella, sage

PEPPERMINT

The mint family is one of the most aromatic and useful plant families, both for herbal medicine, the culinary arts and aromatherapy. Excellent for headaches and cough, peppermint is a stimulant and revitalizer. A derivative, menthol, is used as an important component in the pharmaceutical and tobacco industries. It is one of the best essential oils for Pitta, being cooling to the digestive fires. It has both antiseptic and expectorant qualities so it is useful for the respiratory tract as an inhalation; useful in the mouth as a mouth wash; or added to toothpaste can be healing to gum infections and canker sores. Ten drops added to a bath can have a cooling affect on the body (especially when you get out).

Common name: Peppermint

Family name: Labiatae (Mint)

Botanical name: Mentha Piperita

Dosha effect: P K–, V o

Taste: pungent

PD taste: pungent

Energy: cooling, moisturizing

Actions: diaphoretic, carminative, nervine, stimulant, analgesic, decongestant, antiseptic

Tissues: plasma, blood marrow and nerves, gums, GI, skin

Indications: colds, fever, sore throat, laryngitis, earache, digestive upset, nervous agitation, headache, dysmenorrhea, hepatobiliary disorders, asthma

Warning: can aggravate severe chills and neurasthenia

Usage: compress, lotion, bath, massage oil, toothpaste, gargle, mouth-wash, aroma lamp, spritzer, inhalations, salve

Aroma: fresh, strong, somewhat grassy-minty odor with a deep balsamic-sweet undertone and a sweet, clean dryout note

Mixes well with: clary sage, sage, eucalyptus, lavender, rosemary, and citrus

PETITGRAIN

Petitgrain oil is made by steam distillation of twigs, leaves, and sometimes unripe fruit of the citrus family, including orange, lemon and tangerine. It is mildly reminiscent of Neroli. Coming from the stems and leaves of the plant, it bring a freshness and a strength not found in the fruit. Petitgrain is excellent in a massage oil for muscle spasm and inflamed tissue. It is good for lymphatic drainage and improves all circulation. It can be helpful as a digestive aid and is very grounding and calming to the nervous system. It is uplifting, good for transition, and for keeping the mind clear.

Common name: Petitgrain

Family name: Rutacea

Botanical name: Citrus Aurantium

Dosha effect: P K–, Vo

Taste: bittersweet

PD taste: sweet

Energy: warming

Actions: digestive, stimulant, antispasmodic, clarifying, antidepressant, tonic

Tissues: skin, nerve, digestive

Indications: poor memory, confusion, anxiety, digestive problems, dyspepsia, flatulence, joint problems, pain, circulation problems

Warning: applied to skin, oil may cause discoloration with sun exposure

Usage: aroma lamp, massage oil, inhalation, spritzers

Aroma: pleasant, fresh-flora, sweet odor, reminiscent of orange flowers with a slightly woody-herbaceous undertone, very faint but sweet-floral dryout notes, "bitter" topnotes

Mixes well with: all citrus, angelica, jatamansi, rosewood, dhavana and champa

PINE

The world's largest production of any one essential oil is pine; it is used in paint thinners, paints, varnishes, etc. There are many different varieties of pine. One of the most therapeutic is Swiss pine, the harvest of which is strictly controlled by the Swiss government, with only dead and dying trees allowed to be harvested. It is known to be a stimulant, helping people to be comfortable with any situation. Men like the smell because it reminds them of the outdoors. It helps you feel open and aware, and is good for circulation.

Common name: Pine

Family name: Coniferae Pinaceae (Pine family)

Botanical name: Pinus Alba/and species

Dosha effect: K V–, P+

Taste: bitter, pungent

PD taste: pungent

Energy: healing, drying

Actions: expectorant, diaphoretic, antiseptic

Tissues: skin, blood, plasma, respiratory

Indications: colds, bronchitis, lung problems, sinus, hair loss, depression

Warning: can be a skin irritant

Usage: aftershave, massage oil, lotion, aroma lamp, bath, spray

Aroma: sweet pine wood, somewhat balsamic-anisic odor, increasingly sweet on dry out, with a resinous bitter undertone

Mixes well with: birch, eucalyptus, myrtle, sandalwood, juniper, citrus, jatamansi, vetiver, lavender, cedarwood, citronella, rosewood, oakmoss

ROSE

Light: whenever people ask if I am addicted to using essential oils, I tell them that I suspect that I am, especially to rose. Being addicted to good things, like exercise, healthy foods, and essential oils, is not a bad thing. If neroli is the princess of essential oils, then rose is the queen. Rose is one of the most difficult essential oils to distill, and takes the most raw material, hand picked at great expense, to produce a small amount of oil. Rose has been highly regarded for thousands of years. Often available in absolute (petroleum extracted) form, aromatherapists prefer steamed distilled. The Moroccan variety is slightly different, having a warmer smell and a yellow color in its absolute form. Bulgarian is regarded as the best of those which are steamed distilled, and seems to have a very wide bouquet. Turkish is somewhat flatter but still acceptable and I find the Indian first and second distillation comparable, if not sometimes superior to, the Bulgarian. Being one of the most expensive essential oils, rose is often adulterated for profit. Reputable suppliers test to guarantee the purity of their product; until you develop your nose, knowing who you buy your oil from is your best hope of a pure product. First distillation yields some of the highest, most volatile components that are so light they are easily lost. It is customary to redistill the spent roses a second time; this is usually combined with the first distillation to ground it and prevent it from evaporating, then sold as "first." The third distillation of the same material produces a somewhat less grand product, and "fourth" distillation is best for blends.

Rose gives a sense of security and spiritual attunement. It keeps your heart open and connected to all things. It reduces anger and strengthens liver function. It is a special gift to women and is important in menopause formulas. In skin care it is important because of its astringent and antiseptic nature, and can be especially beneficial for Pitta-type inflammation and skin allergies.

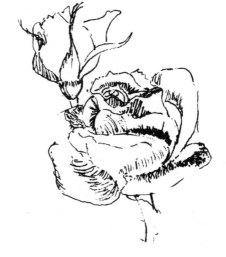

Common name: Rose

Family name: Rosaceae

Botanical name: Rose Damascena/ Centrifolia/others

Dosha effect: V P K=

Taste: bitter, pungent, astringent, sweet

PD taste: sweet

ROSE (continued)

Energy: cooling, moisturizing

Actions: alterative, emmenagogue, refrigerant, nervine, carminative, laxative, astringent, cell regenerator, aphrodisiac, stimulant, antidepressant

Tissues: plasma, blood, marrow, nerve, reproductive, skin, liver, GI

Indications: amenorrhea, dysmenorrhea, uterine hemorrhage, inflamed eyes, dizziness, mental illness, depression, headache, sore throat, enlarged tonsils, impotence, nervousness, grief, aged skin, acne

Warning: restrain use if high Kapha condition is present

Usage: perfumes, lotion, compress, bath, inhalations, massage, diffusers, all uses

Aroma: *rosa damascena*: warm, deep-floral, slightly spicy and immensely rich, truly reminiscent of red roses, with nuances in spicy and honey-like notes; *rosa centrifolia*: deep-sweet, rich and tenacious floral rose-odor

Mixes well with: sandalwood, jasmine, neroli, lavender, bergamot, clary sage, geranium, patchouli, rosewood

ROSEMARY

Rosemary is another oil that should be in everyone's medicine cabinet. It has almost as many uses as lavender. Roman students studied with garlands of rosemary around their heads, then wore the garlands when they took their exams to help them remember. You can do this today much more easily with just a drop of rosemary on your book or on a handkerchief to use when you study and when you are tested. Added to shampoo and cream rinses, rosemary stimulates circulation for the hair and scalp. It can prevent hair loss, reduce oil build-up, and in combination with sage is reported to stop/prevent gray hair from spreading. It is recommended in treatment of cellulite, along with orange and other oils. It is useful for headaches, tension relief, and clarity. For various types of arthritis, it can be useful in combination with eucalyptus, wintergreen, the melaleuca family and lavender. Eucalyptus and rosemary are standard inhalations for respiratory and sinus problems, and could also be used in nose drops, gargles and for liver - gall bladder problems (including stones). Use two to four drops diluted, two to four times a day.

Common name: Rosemary

Family name: Labiatae

Botanical name: Rosemarinus Officinalis

Dosha effect: K V–, P+

Taste: pungent, bitter

PD taste: pungent

Energy: heating, drying

Actions: diaphoretic, carminative, stimulant, emmenagogue, antiseptic, antispasmodic, cholagogue, cardiotonic, nerve tonic, antidepressant

Tissues: muscle, blood, plasma, skin, nerve, heart, endocrine

Indications: liver ailments, gall bladder inflammation, gallstones, flu, colds, asthma, rheumatism, poor memory, weak ego, blemished skin, dandruff, hair loss, burns, wounds

Warning: do not use during pregnancy or with epilepsy; highly stimulating oil

Usage: inhalation, compress, massage oil, shampoo, conditioner, cooking, aroma lamp, all uses

ROSEMARY (continued)

Aroma: strong, fresh, woody-herbaceous, somewhat minty-forest-like, clean, woody-balsamic bodynote with dry-herbaceous but pleasant tenacious bitter-sweet note

Mixes well with: lavender, citronella, oreganum, thyme, pine, cedarwood, petitgrain, musk, eucalyptus, frankincense, cinnamon

ROSEWOOD

Light: Anyone in the healing or serving professions should not be without this oil. I find this oil grounding and connecting. When used externally in a skin lotion or oil it can help protect from others' energy, and maintain a clean and enclosed aura. It is probably one of the best oils for dry skin and hair. It removes anxiety and fear and is excellent for Vata conditions; it helps people come back in the body. Its warm woody fragrance is an excellent middle note or blend enhancer and can give body to a blend which has too much high or low note.

Common name: Rosewood

Family name: Lauraceae (Laurel)

Botanical name: Aniba Roseodora

Dosha effect: V K–, P+

Taste: sweet, pungent

PD taste: sweet

Energy: warming, moisturizing

Actions: antiseptic, cell regenerative, tonic, alterative, relaxant, euphoric

Tissues: skin, nerve, circulation, blood

Indications: tiredness, nervousness, stress, dry skin, acne, aged skin, headache, nausea, anxiety, sadness, infections

Warning: none

Usage: perfumes, massage oils, lotion, bath, shampoo, diffuser, all

Aroma: refreshing, sweet-woody, somewhat floral-spicy topnote is camphoraceous-peppery, reminiscent of cineole and nutmeg.

Mixes well with: geranium, jatamansi, angelica, sandalwood, dhavana, vetiver, lilac, neroli

SAGE

There are several varieties of sage. We originally used Spanish sage in many of our formulas, and were very pleased with its aroma and the way it blended with other oils. The one time we dried Dalmatian sage, it took over every formula that we had; overwhelming with a very lingering, tenacious top note, reminiscent of mugwort. A member of the mint family, sage can contain up to 50% ketone and so generally is not recommended for internal use. It is instead recommended to use clary sage internally because it has many of the same properties without the toxicity. Used externally, sage has very strong estrogenic properties and can be helpful with hot flashes, water retention, gum infections, and the prevention of wrinkles. It is used to stop the progression of gray hair. Jeanne Rose mentions that it can cause vertigo if it is inhaled to excess.

Common name: Sage

Family name: Labiatae

Botanical name: Salvia Officinalis

Dosha effect: K V–, P+

Taste: pungent, bitter, astringent

PD taste: pungent

Energy: heating, drying

Actions: diaphoretic, expectorant, nervine, astringent, alterative, diuretic, disinfectant, carminative, antispasmodic, stimulant, hypertensor, emmenagogue, antidepressant

Tissues: plasma, blood, nerve, skin, kidneys, heart, immune, endocrine, gums

Indications: colds, flus, sore throat, laryngitis, swollen lymph glands, night sweats, hair loss, nervous dysfunction, dermatitis, dandruff, metabolism, disfunction of adrenocortical glands, anemia, jaundice, hypotension, infertility, gum infections

Warning: abortive and toxic in high doses, high Vata, or in nursing mothers; not for internal use

Usage: lotion, aroma lamp, massage oil, room deodorant, shampoo, conditioner

Aroma: fresh, herbaceous, eucalyptol-camphor like odor, sharp pine-like topnote and little or no sweetness on dry out

Mixes well with: lavender, rosemary, citrus, rosewood, citronella, pine

SANDALWOOD

Along with rosewood, hina, amber and myrrh, sandalwood is one of the five essential oils to put into your metaphysical first aid kit. Light has anointed herself with sandalwood since she was a little girl. Sandalwood helps to keep you grounded, close to your divine essence, helps through periods of fear, and allows you to surrender to divine will. Sandalwood is one the strongest-smelling plants in the world.

When western man first came to Hawaii, the mountains were covered with sandalwood, and it was said you could smell it on the breeze from 20 miles away, before you could even see the land. Sandalwood has important antibacterial properties and is useful as a gargle: one drop sandalwood, one drop cajeput in four ounces water, used as needed. This gargle has been very helpful to Light when she started to come down with a sore throat while traveling through polluted areas of Bombay. Light also uses it in her Tantra classes because it helps reprogram the brain and assists people in redirecting their sexual energy to a spiritual purpose. Sandalwood stimulates the pituitary and pineal glands and is a builder of the entire endocrine system. Very high in substances that are similar to male hormone (androgen). It is the regulator of the uterus and has a history of use with venereal disease.

Common name:	Sandalwood
Family name:	Santalaceae
Botanical name:	Santalum Album
Dosha effect:	P V–, K o
Taste:	bitter, sweet, astringent
PD taste:	sweet
Energy:	cooling, moisturizing
Actions:	alterative, hemostatic, antipyretic, nervine, antiseptic, antibacterial, carminative, sedative, refrigerant, expectorant, elevating, moisturizer, antispasmodic, diuretic, tissue regenerative, aphrodisiac
Tissues:	plasma, blood, muscle, marrow and nerve, reproductive
Indications:	cystitis, urethritis, vaginitis, acute dermatitis, herpes zoster, bronchitis, palpitations, gonorrhea, sunstroke, dry skin, acne, laryngitis, nausea, tuberculosis, depression, insomnia, prostatis, nervousness, anxiety, impotence, egocentricity
Warning:	do not use if high Kapha or severe lung congestion is present

SANDALWOOD (continued)

Usage: perfumes, massage oils, gargle, lotion, bath, inhalations, compresses, douches, diffusers

Aroma: extremely soft, sweet-woody, almost animal-balsamic odor, little or no topnote, uniform and outstanding tenacity

Mixes well with: rose, ylang ylang, rosewood, geranium, jatamansi, vetiver, frankincense, myrrh, tuberose, opoponox, oakmoss, labdanum, patchouli, musk, clove

TANGERINE

Tangerine is an American hybrid of mandarin which is larger and has a milder smell. It is a favorite with children and pregnant women because of its soothing and uplifting qualities. It helps sluggish digestion and relaxes muscle spasm.

Common name: Tangerine

Family name: Rutacea (Rue) Reticulata

Botanical name: Citrus Mandurensis

Dosha effect: V P–, K o

Taste: bitter pungent

PD taste: pungent

Energy: cooling, drying

Actions: refrigerant, carminative, expectorant, diuretic, nervine

Tissues: muscles, GI, nerve, endocrine

Indications: insomnia, rheumatism, PMS, stomach, liver, gall bladder problems, tension, fear, sadness, irritability

Warning: possibly phototoxic (sun action) with exposure

Usage: aroma lamp, diffuser, pillow, massage oil, perfume oil, food and drink

Aroma: fresh, sweet odor, reminiscent of bitter orange; lacking dryness, perfumery notes and amine "fishy" note characteristic of mandarin

Mixes well with: sandalwood, citrus oils, rosewood, cardamon, coriander

TEA TREE

Probably one of the most commonly used essential oils in the U.S., in part due to the Melaleuca Company multi-level marketing, it has a long history of use in holistic care, especially as an anti-fungal agent. It is excellent for skin conditions including insect bite and eczema; in addition it has strong anti-viral properties useful for colds and sore throats, as inhalations and gargles. Tea tree has been studied in both Europe and the United States as a douching treatment for candida albicans. Susanne Fischer-Rizzi recommends 5 drops in one half pint water as a douche, or as a five percent tea tree salve applied to a tampon. She also reports that American studies have shown its effectiveness in this way with trichomoniasis.

Common name: Tea Tree

Family name: Myrtaceae (Myrtle)

Botanical name: Melaleuca Alternifolia

Dosha effect: VPK=

Taste: bitter, pungent, sweet

PD taste: sweet

Energy: cooling, moisturizing

Actions: fungicidal, vulnerary, antiseptic, anti-infection, expectorant, stimulant, antiviral, antibacterial, antipyretic

Tissues: skin, nerves, respiratory

Indications: abscess, acne, herpes, pruritus, dermatitis, dandruff, infectious diseases, urinary infections, asthma, bronchitis, tuberculosis, athlete's foot, candida, fungal infections, ringworm, wounds, insect/spider/scorpion bites

Warning: none

Usage: salve, vaginal douche, inhalations, food and drink, diffusers, bath

Aroma: warm-spicy, aromatic-terpenic (monoterpene of pine) odor, reminiscent of nutmeg, cardamon, and sweet marjoram, strong emphasis on the terpinene and terpineol notes

Mixes well with: lavender, clove, rosemary, geranium, neroli, trifolia, chamomiles, eucalyptus, niaouli

THYME, RED

Thyme is grown world wide in both tropical and temperate climates and is commonly distilled and readily available. There are numerous varieties with differing chemical compositions giving Thyme wide application to numerous physical complaints. Spanish Thyme (vulgaris, zygis and oreganum varieties) is high in thymol and useful in Sungal, yeast, viral and bacterial infections. It's high phenol content demands respect for possible skin irritation. Sometimes known as White Thyme (fresh) or Red Thyme (aged.) Lemon Thyme (hiemalis variety) is high in citral (aldelhides) and is good for skin use. The Geranial Type is high in alcohol's, which makes it good in all uses and is less irritating to the skin. It is useful in female and urinary complaints, the respiratory tract and for skin infections. Thymus mastichina (wild margoram) is especially good for the lungs due to its expectorant qualities (cineol.) Thymus Satureioides is an immune builder, general boost to energy, useful in chronic infections and a reputed aphrodisiac. Caution: skin irritant. (Borneol-carvacral, phenols) All the thyme chemotypes are generally heating and with the lemon and geraniol types, less irritating. Skin irritability can be avoided even in babies by applying several drops to the hard skin on the bottoms of the feet or by adding to massage oil at extreme dilution (1% or less). Always use in moderation due to its great strength.

Common name: Thyme, Red

Family name: Labiatae (Mint)

Botanical name: Thymus Vulgaris

Dosha effect: V K–, P+

Taste: pungent

PD taste: pungent

Energy: heating, moisturizing

Actions: antispasmodic, carminative, antibiotic, antiseptic, stimulant, tonic, antidepressant, analgesic, rubefacient, disinfectant, antiviral

Tissues: respiratory, immune, digestive, nerve

Indications: physical/psychological weakness, neurasthenia, staphylococcus, colds, bronchitis, flu, whooping cough, sinusitis, missing periods, athlete's foot, metabolism, burns, wounds, anemia, debility, acne, dermatitis, insomnia, cystitis, cellulitis, rheumatism

Warning: skin irritant in high concentration; do not use with epileptic conditions, hyperthyroidism, high blood pressure, or during pregnancy

Usage: compress, massage oil, inhalation, food, diffuser, salve

Aroma: rich, powerful, sweet, warm-herbaceous, somewhat spicy and distinctly aromatic

Mixes well with: rosemary, oregano, lemon, orange, bergamot, melissa

TURMERIC

Turmeric has received recent attention because of its energizing effect on the immune system, and is being used in some treatment of AIDS. It is used in cosmetics for oily skin and to cleanse and detoxify. It is a favorite with the food flavoring industry, in part because of its bright yellow color. It has grounding properties, helping you to feel present and in charge. Excellent for confusion and anxiety. There is some indication that use of turmeric helps stabilize blood sugar.

Common name: Turmeric

Family name: Ziniberaceae

Botanical name: Curcuma Longa

Other name: Haridra

Dosha effect: V K–, P+, (V+ in excess

Taste: pungent, bitter, astringent

PD taste: pungent

Energy: heating, moisturizing

Actions: stimulant, alterative, antibacterial, vulnerary, carminative

Tissues: all tissue-elements

Indications: indigestion, poor circulation, cough amenorrhea, pharyngitis, skin disorders, diabetes, arthritis, anemia, wounds, bruises, AIDs (all auto immune diseases)

Warning: do not use in cases of acute jaundice, hepatitis, high Pitta, or pregnancy

Usage: massage oil, facial creams, lotions, compresses, food

Aroma: spicy and fresh, reminiscent of sweet orange, ginger, and galanga; Japanese: warm, dry-woody, powdery, camphoraceous, slightly peppery-spicy with peculiar undertone reminiscent of Atlas cedarwood oil

Mixes well with: in perfumery it has been known to blend with cystus, elecampane, ginger, labdanum, musk

VALERIAN ROOT

Bryan: Valerian oil is an ally in times of pain. Its pungent, strong, animal-like smell can be very helpful for sleepless nights, or to ease aches and pains. In my chiropractic practice in Oregon and Hawaii, we would apply this to the skin and ultrasound it into sore shoulders and necks. When mixed with pleasant-smelling oils that have similar properties, its strong smell is countered and covered. Because of its strength, it is recommended to use small amounts; too much can dull the thought processes. Warning: if pain persists, consult a physician.

Common name: Valerian Root

Family name: Valerianacea

Botanical name: Valeriana Officinalis (Wallichii - Indian, and Oficinalio - European)

Other name: Tagara

Dosha effect: V K–, P+

Taste: bitter, pungent, sweet, astringent

PD taste: pungent

Energy: heating

Actions: nervine, antispasmodic, sedative, carminative

Tissues: plasma, muscle, marrow, nerve

Indications: insomnia, hysteria, delirium, neuralgia, convulsions, epilepsy, vertigo, nervous cough, dysmenorrhea, palpitations, migraine, chronic skin diseases, flatulence, colic, stress, diabetes, stomach problems

Warning: large doses produce paralysis (overly constricts Vata); use in small amounts; avoid absolute form when possible

Usage: massage oil, salve, aroma lamp, tea, drinks, food

Aroma: warm-woody, balsamic-rootlike odor with a distinct animal undertone of musk-like character and great tenacity; topnote: fresh-green, slightly camphoraceous

Mixes well with: eucalyptus, rosemary, lavender, wintergreen, juniper, tea tree, pine, patchouli, petitgrain, cedarwood, oakmoss

VANILLA

Vanilla is commonly available as an oleoresin and occasionally as an essential oil or absolute. Extraction by ethyl alcohol (grain) is necessary if it is to be used internally. Vanilla is mixable in essential oils for blending purposes. The odor is a relaxant for stress, anger, and tension, and it can be added to a blend for aphrodisiac effect for tense lovers.

Common name: Vanilla (Oleoresin)

Family name: Orchidaceae (Orchid)

Botanical name: Vanilla Plantifolia

Dosha effect: V P–, K+ +

Taste: bitter, sweet

PD taste: sweet

Energy: warm, moisturizing

Actions: tonic calms, relaxes, softens anger, frustration, irritability; mild stimulant for menstruation

Tissues: nerve

Indications: anger, frustration, irritability, late periods, supports happiness and joy, as a tonic - stimulant

Warning: none

Usage: cooking, perfume, massage oil, creams, lotions, aroma lamp

Aroma: extremely rich, sweet, somewhat woody and animal (castoreum-like) tobacco-like and very deep in its balsamic, sweet-spicy bodynote

Mixes well with: sandalwood, vetiver, opoponox, spice oils, bergamot, rose

VETIVER

Nothing brings you back to your center as strongly as vetiver. When you feel scattered, the use of vetiver in a blend can end the confusion—your choices suddenly become clear. In India, this grassy plant is sown wherever there is erosion of the soil. Its strong roots hold onto the soil and prevent loss. It is useful for aging or irritated skin. It is reputed to have an aphrodisiac effect and be a female tonic. It helps to connect you to the earth and feel your purpose. It is reported to be useful in post-partum depression.

Common name: Vetiver

Family name: Graminae

Botanical name: Vetiveria Zizanoides

Dosha effect: V–, K P+

Taste: sweet, bitter

PD taste: sweet

Energy: warm, grounding

Actions: antiseptic, tonic, relaxant, woman's hormone balancer, grounding, regenerating, strengthening, aphrodisiac, rubefacient, moth repellent

Tissues: skin, nerve, reproductive, joints

Indications: arthritis, root chakra blockage, nervousness, insomnia, rheumatism, stress, disconnectedness, anorexia, postpartum depression, aging skin, tired skin, irritated menopause, loss of appetite

Warning: in creating a lotion or perfume, it can take over the smell

Usage: lotion, bath, massage oil, patches, perfumes (use small amounts); this is one of the strongest base notes and should never be more than 5% of a blend

Aroma: sweet and very heavy woody-earth, reminiscent of roots and wet soil, rich undertone of "precious wood" notes

Mixes well with: rosewood, jatamansi, all citrus, sandalwood, dhavana, angelica, geranium, ylang ylang, rose, lavender, cinnamon, patchouli, oakmoss and clary sage

WINTERGREEN

Wintergreen smells similar to birch, and because birch is so much more available, it has often been sold as wintergreen. It has wonderful stimulant properties. It has been used traditionally in liniments and salves for muscle spasm. Wintergreen has stimulant, antiseptic, diuretic, and emmenagogue properties. It may be used for boils, swelling, fluid retention, lymphatic congestion, or in a douche for leucorreah. Makes an excellent gargle for a sore throat, and has been used to treat genital infections (douche or sitz bath). A familiar taste in gum, candy, root beer, and toothpaste, the food flavoring industry uses synthetic methyl salicylate.

Common name: Wintergreen

Family name: Heather

Botanical name: Gaultheria Procumbens

Dosha effect: P K–, V o

Taste: pungent

PD taste: pungent

Energy: cooling/moisturizing

Actions: carminative, astringent, analgesic, antiseptic, expectorant, diuretic

Tissues: muscle, skin, reproductive

Indications: muscle pain, rheumatism, sciatica, genital infection

Warning: when using this oil internally, do not use more than one drop

Usage: massage oil, douche, inhalation, aroma lamp

Aroma: intensely sweet-aromatic odor, often displaying a peculiar creamy-fruity topnote and sweet-woody dryout

Mixes well with: anise, calamus, vanilla, lavender, rosemary, sage, birch, fir, mints, juniper, eucalyptus, ylang ylang, tuberose

YLANG YLANG

Ylang Ylang is sold in absolute form; as steam-distilled "extra" (best); "third" (for soap); and "complete oil," a confusing blend of "off" grades and sometimes artificial ingredients, often misrepresented as real. Ylang ylang has an odor that cannot be appreciated except in extreme dilutions. It brings out warmth, self confidence, the feminine side, and sensitivity. A balancer to the female immune system, it reduces tension, cramps, negative emotions, and headaches. It is reported to help with hysteria, high blood pressure, oily skin, aging, and depression.

Common name: Ylang Ylang
Family name: Annonaceae (Custard Apple)
Botanical name: Cananga Odorate
Dosha effect: P V–, K+
Taste: sweet, bitter
PD taste: sweet
Energy: cooling/moisturizing
Actions: sedative, general tonic, antiseptic, aphrodisiac, balancing
Tissues: skin, nerve, reproductive
Indications: high blood pressure, tachycardia, nervous headaches, oily skin, combination skin, aging skin, stressed skin, PMS, fear, rage, anger, low self-confidence, frigidity, impotence, nervous depression, inner coldness
Warning: too much can cause nausea; beware absolute "complete oil"
Usage: perfumes, bath, lotion, massage oil, aroma lamp, diffuser
Aroma: a powerful and intensely sweet, but also balsamic floral, odor; an unusual tenacity in its floral-woody undertone
Mixes well with: rosewood, vetiver, opoponox, bergamot, tuberose, cedarwood

RARE OILS

AJWAN

Light: Ajwan is a wild celery seed in India. While in India, after eighteen hours of travel and with much to do in the smoggy city of Bombay, I found myself with a nervous stomach, experiencing indigestion (what I would now classify as a high Vata condition). Fortunately, one of my first stops was an essential oil supplier, and one of the first oils that he had me smell was ajwan. I immediately felt grounded, connected, and noticed an easing of all my symptoms. Added to food, ajwan can stimulate a poor appetite. Inhaled, it can be beneficial for sinus congestion. Its gift is that it clears out deep-seated congestion and stagnation in both respiratory and digestive tracts.

Common name: Ajwan (Celery Seed)

Family name: Umbelliferae (Carrot)

Botanical name: Apium Graveolens; other - Wild Celery Seed

Dosha effect: K V–, P+

Taste: salty, pungent

PD Taste: pungent

Energy: heating, moisturizing

Actions: stimulant, expectorant, carminative, antispasmodic, lithotrophic (dispels stones)

Tissues: plasma, nerves

Indications: the common cold, bronchitis, respiratory infection, cough, laryngitis, bronchitis, arthritis

Warning: do not use if hyperacid condition is present

Usage: food, tea, steam, massage lotion, gargle

Aroma: pungent, herbaceous and medicinal with a fresh almost green cuminic topnote

Mixes well with: seaweed extract (external use) - dhavana, juniper, eucalyptus, camphor, wintergreen, sandalwood, black pepper, basil

AMBER

Here in the West this oil is used as a base for men's cologne and aftershave because of its leather smell. It is used in India for many religious ceremonies and is composed of a mixture of different essential oils including seasonal variations of styrax, sandalwood, labdanum, and sometimes saffron. The demand is high for this oil and so it is made year-round. The formula varies according to family recipes and the availabilities of the oils. The pure amber portion of the oil blend is steam distilled from the fossilized resin found worldwide. It is very balancing and energizing to the chakras, especially the heart. This oil is calming, energy balancing and protects the wearer from negative influences.

Common name: Amber
Botanical name: Pinus Succinifera
Family name: Pinaceae
Dosha Effect: P V K–
Warning: do not take internally
Usage: perfume, chakra anointment, lotions, salve
Aroma: smoky, tar-like, resinous, like tanned leather

ANGELICA

Good for all dosha types, except Pitta in excess. The Archangel of Healing is embodied in angelica, bringing strength, bravery and perseverance. The plant concentrates its strength in the root and brings the strength and substance of the earth element to us. It is one of the first essential oils we reach for in any infection or immune deficiency. Its tonic nature builds tissue and also brings balance to hormonal excesses or deficiencies. Relative to dong quai, it is a female rejuvenative of note. Susanne Fischer-Rizzi in *Complete Aromatherapy Handbook* recommends nose drops of one drop angelica in four ounces of water as a remedy for nasal polyps. Excellent as inhalation for respiratory problems, added to food or tea for nervous stomach.

Common name: Angelica Root/Seeds

Family name: Umbelliferae (Carrot)

Botanical name: Angelica Officialis/Archangelica

Other name: Choraka - Indian name,
Dong Quai - Chinese relative

Dosha effect: V P K=, P+ (in excess)

Taste: pungent, sweet

PD taste: sweet

Energy: heating and moistening

Actions: stimulant, tonic, emmenagogue, carminative, diaphoretic, expectorant, alterative

Tissues: plasma, blood, muscle, marrow and nerve, (endocrine reproductive)

Indications: amenorrhea, dysmenorrhea, menstrual cramps, PMS, anemia, headaches, colds, flus, arthritis, hiccups, rheumatic pain, poor circulation, adrenal excess

Warning: do not use with hypertension, high Pitta conditions generally (cysts or tumors); use with care during pregnancy; may be phototoxic

Usage: inhalative, nose drops, massage oil, diffuser, tea, as an infusion, tincture

Aroma: light, somewhat peppery topnote, rich, somewhat herbaceous-earthy, woody bodynote, musky-animal-like w/spicy undertone

Mixes well with: rose, immortelle, keawa, St. Johns wort, yarrow, vetiver, rosewood, petitgrain, fennel, eucalyptus, dill, cumin, blue chamomile

BRAHMI

Brahmi is the medicated oil of the gotu kola leaf. It is a common edible groundcover found in much of the tropics, and is said to be the preferred food of the mother elephant during her entire pregnancy. In Ayurveda it is known as the rejuvenator for all systems in the body and is one of the most commonly used medicated oils. It can be found occasionally in a steam distilled form that is quite costly. Brahmi is excellent for hair growth and the prevention of baldness.

Common name: Brahmi
Family name: Umbelliferae
Botanical name: Hydrocotyle Asiatica
Other name: Gotu Kola
Dosha Effect: V P K–
Taste: bitter, sweet
PD taste: sweet
Energy: cooling and moistening
Actions: nervine, tonic, alterative, rejuvenative
Tissues: all tissues
Indications: hair loss, muscle spasms, skin conditions
Warning: in sensitive individuals may aggravate itchiness of the skin
Usage: massage oil, conditioner, shampoo
Aroma: sweet, fruity, medicinal but fresh herbal smell
Mixes well with: sandalwood

CASSIA

This essential oil contains medicinal qualities similar to cinnamon but its smell is sweeter and more pleasant. The oil is used to give colors to many perfume blends. In certain areas the primitive distillation apparatus, still used, contains copper piping which gives a red tone to the oil. Rare because it comes from China and Vietnam.

Common name: Cassia

Botanical name: Cinnamomum Cassia

Family name: Lauracea

Other name: Canela

Dosha Effect: V K–, P+

Taste: sweet and astringent

PD taste: sweet

Energy: heating

Action: stimulant, circulatory enhancer

Tissues: blood, circulatory

Indications: vomiting, gastritis, irritation, headaches

Warning: too much can be irritating to the skin

Usage: flavoring, massage oils, perfumes, lotions, aroma lamps

Aroma: intensely sweet with a somewhat balsamic undertone

Mixes well with: cardamon, fennel, orange, bergamot

CHAMPA

Champa absolute is a rare material most often made from concrete (ether extraction), commonly co-distilled with sandalwood as an attar, and available locally, where produced, as a medicated oil. Steam-distilled essential oil is rare, costly, and unfortunately does not well represent the flower's smell. All forms of production are known for the sweet floral smell. Grown in the same areas as ylang ylang, champa is frequently adulterated with it, and many poor imitations are offered on the market. It has aphrodisiac qualities and can transport you to an enlightened point of reference. It is useful for irritated skin.

Common name: Champa

Family name: Michelia Champaca

Botanical name: Apocynaceae - Magnolia

Other Name: Champaca, Plumeria, Frangapani

Dosha effect: P K–, V+ (in excess)

Taste: sweet, bitter, pungent

PD taste: pungent

Energy: cooling, moisturizing

Actions: emollient, antipyretic, aphrodisiac

Tissues: skin, reproductive

Indications: frigidity, skin irritation

Warning: absolute: avoid internal use and do not use at all during pregnancy

Usage: aroma lamp, diffuser perfume oil, massage oil

Aroma: delicately floral, delightfully sweet, reminiscent of neroli, ylang, ylang, with some notes which recall clary sage

Mixes well with: rose, violet, sandalwood, rosewood, jasmine, cypress, lotus, vetiver

CYPERUS

This oil has a way of making me feel warm, open and creative. It is made from a grass that grows wild in India, and as more people smell and experience it, it will be requested more often.

Common name: Cyperus

Family name: Cyperacea

Botanical name: Cyperus Rotundus

Other name: Cypriol - Nagar Mustaka

Dosha effect: P K V–

Taste: bitter, sweet

PD taste: sweet

Energy: heating, drying

Actions: astringent, alterative, expectorant, sedating and calming to the mind

Tissues: skin, muscle, plasma, respiratory

Indications: diarrhea, skin rashes, tonic, excess bleeding

Usage: massage oil, compress, gargle, suppositories, perfumes, basti (enema)

Aroma: woody, spicy and sweet with rich undertones of the earth

Mixes well with: labdanum, bergamot, sandalwood, vetiver, sage clary, patchouli

DHAVANA

Dhavana is somewhat a rare oil in the West although it appears to be used by the food flavoring industry, with rumors having Snapple® being a major user. Used in many pancha karma clinics in India for ovarian and uterine cysts, both as a compress and a douche. Excellent for menopausal women and useful in regulating and balancing menstruation. A very strong-smelling oil; always use in small amounts and dilute well. Many people feel it has an interesting strawberry-like undertone.

Common name: Dhavana
Family name: Compositae
Botanical name: Artemisia Pallens
Other name: Davana
Dosha effect: P V K–
Taste: sweet, bitter
PD taste: sweet
Energy: warm
Actions: antiseptic, aphrodisiac, nervine, heart
Tissues: muscle, blood, circulatory, reproductive tissue
Indications: gout, skin irritation, anger, energy balancing, ovarian cysts
Warning: always dilute before using internally
Usage: douche, patches, compress, massage oil, food
Aroma: sharp, penetrating, bitter-green, foliage-like and powerfully herbaceous with a sweet, balsamic, tenacious undertone.
Mixes well with: clary sage, sandalwood, lavender, geranium, labdanum, oakmoss, yarrow

ELECAMPANE

Light: This oil is probably one of the most rejuvenating oils for the respiratory system. Victoria Edwards told me that she had some clients that were respiratory therapists and were having very good results using it. At one time I had a bad tooth which caused sinus infection that drained into my nasal cavity. I used this essential oil with good results. It is not readily available and is quite costly in both absolute and steam-distilled form.

Common name: Elecampane

Family name: Compositae

Botanical name: Inula Graveolens

Dosha effect: K V–, P+

Taste: sweet, bitter, pungent

PD taste: pungent

Energy: warming, drying

Actions: expectorant, nervous system tonic, rejuvenative, galactagogue

Tissues: lung, upper respiratory,

Indications: colds, bronchial congestion, cough, lung infection

Warning: can be irritating to the skin and the mucous membranes in direct contact; not for internal use

Usage: recommend inhalations only; best in inhalation or in dilute amounts in perfumes, massage oils and lotions

Aroma: woody, sweet, honey-like, root-like, with a fatty undertone

Mixes well with: rosemary, labdanum, lavender, tuber rose, cedarwood, violet, olibanum, cinnamon, patchouli, musk, and frankincense

GALBANUM

The essential oil is made from the oleogum resin of a member of the carrot family. It is used extensively in the perfume industry and historically as an incense and healing agent. Used externally for wound healing, skin inflammation, arthritic pain and female problems. Used psychologically to balance extremes or intense emotion.

Common name: Galbanum

Family name: Umbelliferae

Botanical name: Ferula Species

Dosha effect: V P K= (V+ in excess)

Taste: bitter, astringent, pungent

PD taste: pungent

Energy: cooling, drying

Actions: astringent, antibiotic, decongestant, emmenagogue, nervine

Tissues: respiratory, endocrine, skin, lymph, joints

Indications: PMS, menopause, lymph, congestion, arthritis, infections, wounds, colds, hysteria, paranoia, anger, flu

Warning: typically used externally

Usage: inhalation, salve, massage oil, liniment, patch

Aroma: intensely green, fresh, leafy odor with a dry woody undertone of balsamic, bark-like character

HINA/HENNA

Hina is another somewhat uncommon Indian oil, often distilled with sandalwood as an attar. The pure oil is not readily available; it is most often found as a blend. It's used in India for religious ceremonies, prayers and to create connectedness or attunement. It is excellent for devotion, for opening psychic abilities and clairvoyance. The herb is used for dying hair, making it red and lustrous and promoting growth. It is the main ingredient of a formula called Shamana used by many Gurus. Swami Muktananda is always remembered by the smell of hina, and it is still used by his followers.

Common name: Hina/Henna

Family name:　Lythraceae

Botanical name: Lawsonia Inermis

Dosha effect:　K V–, P+

Taste:　sweet, bitter

PD taste:　sweet

Energy:　warming/moisturizing

Actions:　opening of psychic, rejuvenative, relaxant, clarity of mind, third eye activator

Tissues:　skin, nails

Indications:　mental disorders, anger, frustration

Warning:　no warning, but traditionally used externally

Usage:　bath, inhalation, massage oil, anointing chakras, meditation

Aroma:　woody, rich, warm, spicy, medicinal, with a leafy undertone, phenolic

Mixes well with: sandalwood, oud, rose, jatamansi

HOPS

This oil can be found in steam-distilled (which is best for aromatherapy) or absolute form. It is used as a fresh plant in brewing beer. The oil can be used for nursing mothers to help with relaxation and for the sleepless nights. In a diffuser mix with lavender, one drop of each. It is important that this oil not be overused.

Common name: Hops

Family name: Moraceae

Botanical name: Humulus Lupulo

Dosha effect: P K V+

Taste: bitter, pungent

PD taste: pungent

Energy: cooling, moisturizing

Actions: nervine, diuretic, febrifuge, carminative

Tissues: nerve, GI, kidney

Indications: fevers, insomnia, migraines

Warning: too much can put you in a stupor; do not prolong the use of this oil for a long period

Usage: massage oil, perfumes, tea

Aroma: the odor is fresh, rich, spicy, sweet and heavy, but very pleasant

Mixes well with: chamomile, lavender, rosemary, lemongrass, angelica

IMMORTELLE

When Light and I were traveling in Morocco, we came across an herb that we had never seen before. We were able to identify it as immortelle and I very quickly gathered half a bushel, took it back to our room and braided it into a garland almost 15 feet long. I hung it over the back of our bed and the rich smell permeated the whole room. Warm and spicy, almost curry-like, it seemed almost magical. Every night we had very vivid, lucid dreams. We carried that garland with us as we traveled through Europe and continued hanging it over our bed, having the most incredible dreams. When it was fully dried, we cut it up and Light used it in her menopausal tea formula. I can't wait to get back to Morocco and pick more (October is the month).

Immortelle is probably one of the most powerful oils for the lymphatic system and the endocrine system. It helps to balance and restore organs to their function. Its a wonderful addition to a skin lotion because it helps with inflammation and acne. Its very helpful in reabsorbing scar tissue and in use with mature skin.

Common name:	Immortelle
Family name:	Compositae (Sunflower family)
Botanical name:	Helichrysum Angustifolium and Orientale
Dosha effect:	V P K=
Taste:	pungent, sweet bitter
PD taste:	sweet
Energy:	heating, moisturizing
Actions:	alterative, antispasmodic, stimulant, antibacterial, antiviral, anti-inflammatory, expectorant, grounding, emmenagogue, nutritive tonic
Tissues:	skin, endocrine system, lymphatic
Indications:	skin allergies, chronic dermatitis, eczema, psoriasis, stomach cramps, gall bladder infection, liver weakness, menstrual cramps, colds, bronchitis, cough, sinus infection, acne, inflamed skin
Warning:	none
Usage:	lotion, compress, perfumes, cosmetics, aftershave, bath, massage oil, lotion, after-sun lotion
Aroma:	powerful and diffusive, pleasant and rich, topnotes so sweet and honey-like as to be overwhelming; sweet-fruity and tea-like delicate undertone is unique and tenacious
Mixes well with:	rock rose, herbanum, bergamot, cypress, angelica, juniper, sandalwood, vetiver, and all citrus

IRIS ABSOLUTE

Light: I love it when I travel through the Southwest and see this wonderful flower blooming all over the mountainsides. I have this feeling of celestial contentment. Iris is reported to be excellent for meditation and clearing your mind. The oil is currently extracted with solvent and is quite expensive. It is very rare and hard to find and is only used in very expensive perfumery.

Common name:	Blue Flag
Family name:	Iridacea
Botanical name:	Iris Versicolor
Other name:	Calamas
Dosha effect:	PK-V+
Taste:	sweet
Energy:	cold
Actions:	alterative, detoxifying, the root is a nutritive tonic
Tissues:	endocrine, excretory, digestive
Indications:	adrenal insufficiency, stomach aches, back problems, diarrhea
Warning:	Do not use during pregnancy
Usage:	best used in perfumes only
Aroma:	sweet, light, fresh
Mixes well with:	rose, neroli, champa, sandalwood

JATAMANSI

Jatamansi has a very strong smell, but one that grows on you, and is an especially useful base oil in a blend. Also known as spikenard, it has been a valued oil since ancient times. In the New Testament, Mary Magdalene used an entire year's income to purchase a small quantity of spikenard for Jesus. At the Last Supper, she massaged his feet and anointed his head with it. When his disciples protested her close contact, Jesus vigorously defended her.

Jatamansi is one of the best oils for calming the nerves. It is grounding for Vata; assisting in controlling the nerves and an out-of-balance mind. In India it is known to be a post-digestive oil. One drop taken near the end of the meal with food or drink calms the stomach. It is a stimulant to the male hormonal system, and brings courage and power. It contains very strong grounding elements, helping people to feel in charge of their lives. It is preserving to mature skin, giving youthfulness and moisture. Jatamansi is excellent for circulation, helping to regulate the heart.

Common name:	Jatamansi
Family name:	Aralia
Botanical name:	Araka Racemosa
Other name:	Spikenard
Dosha effect:	K V–, P+
Taste:	sweet, pungent
PD taste	sweet
Energy:	warming, moisturizing
Actions:	expectorant, nutritive tonic, sedative, alterative, demulcent of internal organs
Tissues:	skin, reproductive, endocrine, digestive
Indications:	menopause, digestion, hormonal stimulant for men
Warning:	too much can dull the brain
Usage:	cosmetic, skin care, perfumes, bath, patches, compress, massage oil, food
Aroma:	heavy, sweet, woody and spicy-animal odor reminiscent of valerian, ginger, cardamon, and atlas cedarwood
Mixes well with:	dhavana, champa, angelica, clary sage, geranium, yarrow, patchouli, cajeput, cedarwood, labdanum, lavender, oakmoss, pine, vetiver, ginger, cardamon

KANCHAMARA OIL
(Honeysuckle - Lonicera Camprifolium)

Kanchamara is an excellent tonic for the female organs and a sexual stimulant-aphrodisiac. Highly regarded in tantra. Honeysuckle was a favorite and familiar smell in Bryan's childhood. He remembers biting off the end of the blossoms and sucking the honey, sometimes pulling the stamen all the way through from the back and bringing out a drop of sweet nectar. It is unfortunate that this is only available in an absolute form, because it would be wonderful in food if it were steam distilled. Most of what is available in the market is actually a synthetic because the oil is quite costly, but the oil absolute is available to perfumers. The smell is nauseatingly honey-like, reported to be aphrodisiac, calming and soothing to the mind.

Common name:	Honeysuckle
Family name:	Caprifoliacea
Botanical name:	Lonicerea camprifolium
Other name:	Chinese Ju Yin Hua
Dosha effect:	PK-V+
Taste:	sweet
Energy:	cooling
Actions:	expectorant, detoxifying, diuretic
Tissues:	lung, circulatory, urinary
Indications:	kidney stones, lung congestion, diabetes, kidney, blood pressure
Warning:	Do not take internally
Usage:	perfumes, bath, cosmetics, compress, massage oil, inhalation
Aroma:	honey-like sweetness
Mixes well with:	citrus, keawa, rosewood, geranium, neroli

KEAWA

This is another one of the wonderful attars of India where the large flowers, weighing up to six ounces each, are steam distilled with sandalwood or other perfume oils to produce an attar. A medicated oil is often prepared with the crushed flowers and sesame seed oil. The steam distillation produces such a small amount of very easily lost distillate that the most common form of production involves hydrocarbon extraction, producing first a concrete and then an absolute. In India keawa is used in religious ceremonies, especially for grieving the dead. It helps with attachment and letting go of anger and resentment. It is used in Ayurvedic medicine for allergies and spleen disorders; helps self esteem, attuning with the divine will of God, and is recommended for transition.

Common name: Keawa

Family name: Pandanaceae

Botanical name: Pandanus Odoratissimus

Other name: Puakinikini (Hawaii), Kewda, Keora

Dosha effect: P K–, V+ (in excess)

Taste: sweet, bitter

Energy: cooling/moisturizing

Actions: calmative, nervine, tonic (nutritive), immune builder, blood tonic

Tissues: muscle, blood

Indications: liver or gall bladder distress; grieving

Warning: do not take internally, most often an absolute

Usage: perfume, lotion, massage oil, bath, massage, anointment of third chakra

Aroma: very sweet, hyacinth-honey-like short topnote of faint, sweet-floral, fresh tone-out

Mixes well with: angelica, rosewood, lavender, myrrh, rose, lilac, styrax, galbanum, clary sage, bergamot, ylang ylang

LOTUS
(Nelumbo Nucifera)

Buddha considered this flower sacred because of its many medical gifts. The flower opens, beckoning the mind into stillness, meditation and unfoldment. The oil works wonders on irritated skin; it is cooling and highly astringent. Also considered sacred by the Hindus, an oil can be made from the seed, the root, and of course a very exquisite perfume made from the petals. It increases clarity, devotion, prosperity and is extremely opening to the heart chakra. This oil is beloved by the goddess Lachmy, giver of prosperity. Lotus is good for headaches and vomiting and can be used for morning sickness and nausea. Rare and expensive, highly prized. (P V–, K+)

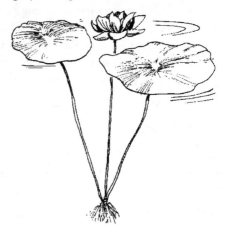

MAGNOLIA ABSOLUTE
(Magnolia Grandiflora)

This is another very expensive oil to produce and is made by some of the finest distilleries in Europe. Steffen Arctander relates that its popularity has been exploited by the perfume industry, with much adulteration and imitation. A few drops of the essential oil is enhancing to self-esteem, is antidepressant, and helpful for anyone quitting a habit, such as smoking. It can be helpful in lowering fevers and rheumatic joints. It has been used in a compress for constipation. Mixes well with champa, rose, sandalwood, geranium and clary sage.

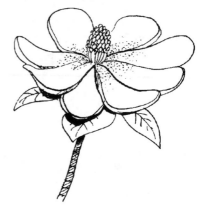

Family name:	Magnoliacea
Botanical name:	Magnolia Officinalis or Magnolia Grandiflora
Other name:	Chinese Hou Po
Dosha effect:	VK-P+
Taste:	sweet
Energy:	sweet
Actions:	carmative, nervine, expectorant
Tissues:	lung, excretory, digestive, urinary tract
Indications:	cramps, to stop smoking, relieves gas, loss of appetite, vomiting, diarrhea, lung infections
Usage:	perfumes, cosmetics, bath soap, massage oil
Aroma:	light, fresh, creamy, elevating, enchanting to the spirit
Mixes well with:	rose, champa, geranium, rosewood, bergamot, jasmine, mogra

Monographs

MOGRA
(Murraya Paniculatta)

During Light's childhood she would occasionally have these flowers braided into her hair, making her feel happy and alive. The flowers are used in celebrations and festivities in India. If you have spent any time in India it is familiar to you because it is sold on every street corner and all around temples and places of devotion. The oil is used in China and Indonesia for the making of perfumes, and is rarely seen in this country. Recently a friend came back from India bearing a gift of one-quarter ounce of this oil and I treasure it like gold. The smell is deep sweet spicy with sour undertones. The dried flowers are sometimes added to tea to add a special fragrance. Occasionally available as a concrete, absolute, or essential oil.

Common name:	Curry patta
Family name:	Rutacea
Botanical name:	Murraya paniculatta
Dosha effect:	Pk-V+
Taste:	sweet, bitter
Energy:	cooling
Actions:	digestive, hair tonic, excretory, diaphoretic
Tissues:	skin, hair
Indications:	fever, insect bites, gray hair, hair loss
Warning:	Excessive use can cause nausea
Usage:	perfumes, bath soap, compress
Aroma:	sweet, refreshing
Mixes well with:	sandalwood, keawa, rosewood, saffron

MUSK, FLORAL

Musk is used in almost all Indian perfumes as a stabilizer, base note, and an extender for the lighter essential oils which are added to it. It is excellent for aphrodisiac formulas. Distilled from the seeds of a variety of Hibiscus, it is very thick and clear. It is an environmentally conscious alternative to the use of musk from musk deer. The practice of killing the animal has almost eradicated the species, although it is possible to extract the musk sacs without killing the animal.

Common name: Musk, Floral

Family name: Malvaceae

Botanical name: Abelmoschus Moschatus

Other name: Veggie musk

Dosha effect: P V K–

Taste: sweet

Energy: warming, moisturizing

Actions: strengthening, eroticizing, refreshing, opening

Tissues: skin

Indications: frigidity, impotence, stagnation

Warning: beware of absolute form

Usage: perfumes, bath, body lotion, aftershave, massage oil

Aroma: rich sweet, floral-musky with a distinct wine-like odor

Mixes well with: jasmine, geranium, rose, champa, ylang ylang, lemon, sandalwood, bergamot, coriander

OAKMOSS

This oil is mostly used by perfumers. The odor is so strong that in making this oil the equipment cannot be used for production of anything else. It is valued because of its fixative qualities, erotic, balancing and calming effects in blends.

Common name: Oakmoss

Family name: Usneaceae

Botanical name: Evernia Furfuracea

Dosha effect: V P K–

Taste: not for internal use

Energy: warming

Actions: sedative, calming, aphrodisiac

Tissues: nerves, skin

Indications: stress, frigidity

Warning: do not take internally, extracted with solvent

Usage: perfumes, lotions

Aroma: very dry, woody, earth-like, bark-like, with a leather-like undertone

OUD

Oud is one of the most highly priced oils in the world. Another name is agar oil. This oil is made only from older agar trees which have been invaded by a fungus. It is used in India and ceremonially by the Arabs and Japanese for anointing the dead and to assist in the transition to the afterlife. Eastern peoples believe that upon death the soul can be "lost" for a period of time. This can be avoided by anointing the person (and close relatives) to create a connection so that the relatives can guide the deceased during this critical period of time.

Bryan: Our partner in California is named Alicia. Her father passed after a long illness, and near the end she was fortunate to be with him and anoint him with a combination of oud and rose. Very soon after his passing he began to appear to her, requesting readings from certain spiritual books. It made sense that this information would be critical to him during transition. She began to take a period of time every day, as much as an hour, to read to him, and converse. We thought that she was a little under stress from his passing and highly imaginative.

Light and Alicia needed to go find bottles, and Alicia said she couldn't go because she had to read to her dad. Light requested that she bring her book and read to her dad in the car (since spirit can travel wherever it wants, shouldn't be a problem). Alicia asked, Dad said fine, and off they went—Light disbelieving—until she heard Alicia's father say, "Thank you Light for bringing me along." This startled her so much that she had to pull off the road. Alicia, we apologize for disbelieving.

Light was teaching a class with me and she accidentally anointed herself with oud thinking it was her beloved rose. For a few minutes she went blank, standing in front of the classroom, and I had to sit her down and take over the lecture. Light recovered, joined in, and on the next break she reported that everyone in the lecture hall had turned into her second grade classmates. She had regressed back to a time when she was asked to read in front of the classroom, and froze. We are careful in our use of oud.

The smell of oud is sweet-sour-rich woody, almost balsamic. This oil is used in fine Oriental perfumes. A drop is used in Indian betel tobacco.

OUD (continued)

Common name: Oud

Family name: Agarwood

Botanical name: Aquilaria Agallosha

Other name: Agar Oil

Dosha effect: V P K=

Taste: sweet, astringent

Energy: warming, balancing

Actions: energy purifying and balancing, relaxant, rejuvenative, transformative, clairvoyant, transcending

Tissues: all tissues

Indications: none

Warning: do not use when public speaking or driving a car

Usage: anointing chakras, inhalation

Aroma: rich and sweet-woody, almost balsamic odor like styrax with a sweetness similar to sandalwood

Mixes well with: rose, geranium, champa, cyperus, sandalwood, vetiver, rosewood, lavender and musk

OUD MUSK BLEND

Bryan: This is a blend containing vegetable musk, oud and some other components, and is a more affordable way to experience oud. The blend is made in attar form where several oils are distilled together to create a less expensive oil at a more affordable price, and a wonderful blended smell. The oil combines the properties of the raw materials, creating and strengthening an elevating effect on the nervous system. I love to use this oil when teaching; it gives me a sense of security and the words seem to come to my mind very clearly. I feel connected as if my speech comes directly from a divine source. Almost like putting my ego to the side and letting the God-self come through.

Common name: Oud Musk

Dosha effect: Good for all doshas

Taste: sweet and bitter

PD taste: sweet

Energy: warming, moistening

Actions: similar to oud and floral musk

Tissues: good for all tissues, used in small amounts

Warning: can be overpowering to the psyche

Usage: perfumes, massage oils, compress, soap, aroma lamp

Aroma: deep, warm, rich, sweet, exotic, spicy and faintly flowery

Mixes well with: geranium, rose, champa, dhavana and jatamansi

SAFFRON

Steam-distilled saffron can be one of the most expensive essential oils on the market and is not generally available. More commonly available is the medicated oil of saffron, having a weaker but pleasant effect. It's similar to sandalwood in that it has properties to balance the nervous system. It promotes digestion and quietness of the mind. It is a rejuvenator to all the tissues of the body.

Common name: Saffron

Family name Iridacea

Botanical name: Crocus Sativus

Other name: Nagakeshara (Indian)

Dosha effect: V P K=

Taste: pungent, bitter, sweet

PD Taste: sweet

Energy: cooling, moisturizing

Actions: alterative, emmenagogue, aphrodisiac, rejuvenative, stimulant, carminative, antispasmodic

Tissues: all tissue elements, especially blood

Indications: menstrual pain and irregularity, menopause, impotence, infertility, anemia, enlarged liver, hysteria, depression, neuralgia, lumbago, rheumatism, cough, asthma, chronic diarrhea

Warning: do not use during pregnancy (can promote miscarriage); can be narcotic in large doses (do not use more than three drops per day internally)

Usage: food, massage oil, perfume, bath

Aroma: most peculiar, intensely sweet, spicy, floral-aldehydic odor with a slightly fatty-herbaceous undertone

Mixes well with: sandalwood, champa, Himalayan cedarwood, lavender, rose, rosewood, violet, neroli

ST. JOHNS WORT

Historically, St. Johns Wort oil has been a medicated oil, made by gathering the yellow flowers of the plant and soaking them in olive oil for a month, straining and repeating until the olive oil becomes a deep red color. With recent demand, an essential oil has been produced, which is one of the more expensive oils. It is known to be anti-inflammatory, cooling and calming to the skin, and revitalizing to the entire body. Somewhat similar to arnica, it can be used in cases of trauma and shock. The medicated oil was traditionally used for dry skin, cracking, irritation, and joint problems. Jeanne Rose in *The Aromatherapy Book* says it has been useful in treating AIDs.

Common name: St. Johns Wort

Family name: Hyperceae

Botanical name: Hypericum Perforatum

Dosha effect: P K–, V+

Taste: bitter, astringent sweet

PD taste: sweet

Energy: cooling, moisturizing

Actions: antispasmodic, expectorant, astringent, nutritive tonic, anti-inflammatory

Tissues: skin, nerve, immune, endocrine

Indications: spinal problems, skin problems, joint pain, ageing, trauma, eczema

Warning: none

Usage: massage lotion, salve, compress

Aroma: "The penetrating smell can be felt as a warm pleasant relaxed feeling, traveling from the nose to the brain." Kurt Schnaubelt

Mixes well with: chamomiles, angelica, yarrow, rosewood

SAVORY

Savory is not commonly used in aromatherapy, but it is used extensively by the food industry. It is very good for obstructed Vata, strengthens the nervous system, relieves flatulence and abdominal pain. It helps the blood tissues hold onto minerals. Because it is so energizing, Susanne Fischer-Rizzi recommends its use for hearing loss: 2 drops savory, 1 teaspoon St. Johns wort medicated oil, applied to a cotton ball and inserted into the outer ear overnight. Similar to thyme in intensity.

Common name: Savory

Family name: Labiatae (Mint)

Botanical name: Satureia Hortensis

Dosha effect: K V–, P+

Taste: pungent

PD taste: pungent

Energy: warming, drying

Actions: stimulant, carminative, astringent, antiseptic

Tissues: digestive, nerve

Indications: abdominal pain, flatulence, diarrhea, insect bites, hearing loss

Warning: always dilute well; may cause irritation; no more than three drops per day

Usage: cooking, perfumes

Aroma: fresh medicinal spicy, reminiscent of sage or thyme, but with a sharpness recalling cumin; dryout is phenolic-harsh.

Mixes well with: thyme, oregano, St. Johns wort, sage, pine, lavender, rosemary

SEAWEED ABSOLUTE

Feecus Versicula is extracted with hydrocarbons and is best used in a perfume blend, although it can be a stimulation for the thyroid and parathyroid. In perfumery, its tenacious smell makes it impossible to use the extraction equipment for any other purpose. Seaweed absolute can be made from almost any seaweed, although Irish moss is most common.

Dosha effect:	V K P+
Taste:	salty, bitter
Energy:	warming, moisturizing
Action:	alterative, soothing, increases tissue growth, moisturizing
Tissues:	endocrine system
Indications:	thyroid, weight problems
Warning:	do not take internally
Usage:	perfume, bath, compress, massage oil
Aroma:	herbaceous, phenolic, woody and dry; odor is reminiscent of the salt and the surf at the beach
Mixes well with:	oakmoss, patchouli, cedarwood, lavender, floral musk and pine

SHAMAMA

Shamama is a blend of essential oils used for meditation and opening the third eye. There are many different formulations; the best mixture is henna, sandalwood and saffron. This blend has wonderful rejuvenative properties, and is excellent as a relaxant. It helps clear anger and frustration, clearing the psychic senses.

STYRAX

Styrax is made from the sap-resin, collected and distilled in Asia Minor and nearby islands. It is reported to have similar uses to benzoin. In an interview, Stevie Wonder reported that he used Asiatic styrax to help maintain his voice. Used in making amber and shamama blends, it can be helpful for improving memory.

Common name: Styrax

Botanical name: Liquidamber Orientalis

Other names: Asian Styrax

Dosha effect: P K–, V+

Taste: astringent, sweet

PD taste: sweet

Energy: cooling, drying

Actions: expectorant, carminative, brain stimulant, tonic, alterative

Tissues: lung, cerebral cortex, olfactory nerve

Indications: sore throat, mental clarity

Warning: do not use too much as it could be overpowering; it is often found in absolute form, so do not take internally unless you are sure it is steam distilled

Aroma: rich, balsamic, sweet, floral, somewhat spicy, reminiscent of lilac, often contains a very strong top note of a hydrocarbon nature (gasoline-like due to the styrene content)

Mixes well with: violet, lavender, rose and champa, ylang ylang, jasmine

TAGETES

Closely related to marigold (calendula), this species is steam-distilled to produce a thick, dark, strong-smelling oil which is softening to any hardened tissue such as scars, calluses, rough skin, etc. It is reported to help the body absorb bunion formation when applied twice daily for one year with concurrent use of a "toe wedge" to help straighten the big toe involved. An important ingredient in skin care for dry, scaly, chapped, cut, scraped or healing skin.

Common name: Tagetes

Family name: Compositae

Botanical name: Tagetes Patula or Glandulifera

Other name: Indian Marigold

Dosha effect: V K–, P+ (in excess)

Taste: bitter, pungent

PD taste: pungent

Energy: heating, moisturizing

Actions: vulnerating, antispasmodic, alterative

Tissues: skin, joints

Indications: skin problems, hard tissue, bunions, cuts, scratches

Warning: sometimes in absolute form

Usage: salve, massage oil, skin creme, perfume oil

Aroma: strongly herbaceous, somewhat sharp with a fruity top note in fresh oil, replaced by a somewhat strange smell: pleasant to some, disagreeable to others

Mixes well with: lavender, jasmine, gardenia, violet, sandalwood

TARRAGON

In Europe it is known as Dragon or Estragon and is another one of the wonderful oils for Vata conditions because it strengthens the nervous system, helps the digestive tract, builds up the immune system, grounds the body, and gives courage to the mind. It is excellent for food flavorings in soups, salads, dressings and sauces. Dr. Valnet speaks of using it for malignant conditions such as cancer and tumors.

Common name: Tarragon

Family name: Compositae

Botanical name: Artemesia Dracunculus

Dosha effect: K V–, P+

Taste: bitter, pungent

PD taste: pungent

Energy: heating, drying

Actions: emmenagogue, diuretic, carminative, antispasmodic, balances autonomic nervous system, vermifuge, digestive stimulant, antiseptic, heart tonic

Tissues: nerve, skin, digestive, blood, immune

Indications: digestive and intestinal spasms, dyspepsia, hiccups, aerophagia, fermentation, parasites, physical weakness, immune system, irregular periods, blood circulation, rheumatism

Warning: do not take when pregnant

Usage: massage oil, bath, compress, inhalation

Aroma: sweet-anisic, green-spicy, slightly celery-like odor, similar to smell of the fresh herb

Mixes well with: cyperus, anise, fennel, dill, lilac, lavender, vanilla, cinnamon, oakmoss and floral bases

TRIFOLIA

Light: This oil is produced from the fruit of a Himalayan variety of prickly ash. It is used in Ayurvedic medicine for constipation. I was introduced to this oil by my Indian teacher (who is 110 years young this year); he had it distilled especially for me because of my tendency to constipation when I travel. It is very effective applied externally to the abdomen. It is also useful for yeast problems in the GI tract when taken internally, and for skin infection, externally. When using this in a blend, begin with a small amount, because it can be very overpowering. It is grounding, warming, mind-clearing and centering. It brings a fresh, clean note to blends.

Common name: Trifolia
Family name: Rutacea (Rue)
Botanical name: Xanthozylum Alatum
Other name: Tumru or "Chinese Wild Pepper"
Dosha effect: VK–, P+
Taste: pungent, sweet
PD taste: sweet
Energy: warming, moisturizing
Actions: antiseptic, antifungal, analgesic
Tissues: plasma, digestive, nerve
Indications: constipation, yeast infection, parasites
Warning: do not use when there is inflammation, swelling or diarrhea
Usage: compress, massage, oil, aroma lamp, lotion
Aroma: warm-woody, green-peppery, spicy odor, reminiscent of cubeb, guaiacwood, faint resemblance to wild roses; deep-floral dryout
Mixes well with: lavender, geranium, cinnamon, clove bud, rosewood, bergamot, sandalwood

TUBEROSE - ABSOLUTE

Another very expensive ($10,000+ per pound) and often adulterated essential oil, it takes 3,600 pounds of flowers to make one pound of absolute. It can be appreciated only in dilution. Being an absolute, its therapeutic applications are limited to external use.

Common name:	Tuberose - Absolute
Family name:	Valerianacea
Botanical name:	Polyanthes Tuberosa
Family name:	Amaryllidaceae
Dosha effect:	V K–, P+
Taste:	sweet, pungent
PD taste:	sweet
Energy:	cooling, moisturizing
Actions:	antidepressant, mood elevator
Tissues:	muscle, skin, nerve
Indications:	stressful situations when you must pay close attention to another's needs
Warning:	do not take internally
Usage:	fine perfumes, bath, massage oils, aroma lamp
Aroma:	a heavy floral, almost nauseatingly sweet, heavy and somewhat spicy odor, reminiscent of honeysuckle, Peru balsam, orange flower absolute, ylang ylang residue fractions, stephanotis flowers
Mixes well with:	opoponox, rosewood, citruses, sandalwood, patchouli

VIOLET LEAF ABSOLUTE

At one time violet flower absolute was expensive but available; now it is even more expensive, and difficult to find. Violet leaf absolute is used for troubled skin and reportedly for throat cancer. Used for the throat chakra, nervous conditions, extremes of emotion, it is calming and relaxing.

Common name: Violet Leaf Absolute

Family name: Violaceae

Botanical name: Viola Odorata

Dosha effect: P K–, V+

Taste: bitter, astringent, pungent

PD taste: pungent

Energy: cooling, moisturizing

Actions: astringent, diaphoretic

Tissues: skin, nervous system

Indications: troubled skin, wounds, fine perfume production

Warning: avoid internal use

Usage: perfumes

Aroma: powerful and peculiar green leaf odor with an indisputable delicate floral note, reminiscent of violets in a bouquet

Mixes well with: tuberose, champa, rose, clary sage, tarragon, cumin, basil

YARROW

Bryan: Yarrow is the herb whose stalks are used in casting the *I Ching*. It has been regarded as a sacred and important plant by many cultures. In herbology, it is one of the oils which are known as "heal-alls," because of its many properties. Susanne Fischer-Rizzi in her book *Complete Aromatherapy Handbook*, describes this as a connector—allowing you to keep your head in the heavens and your feet on the ground. The plant itself stands very tall with a thin stalk, its flowers reaching out into the air element and its roots firmly grounded in the earth. It is one of my favorite oils when I need balance; very useful during menopause, especially when nothing else seems to work for emotional upsets. Is excellent for excess bleeding in any circumstance. Very useful for fevers because it is a diaphoretic. It has a bluish-green color because of its high azulene content, and is placed in the chart in the upper right hand corner with blue chamomile. It is known to have anti-phlogistic (fluid moving) and anti-inflammatory qualities due to its high sesquiterpene content. Its a good regulator for the kidneys and the hair. It is one of the immune-building essentials that I reach for whenever I'm feeling sick.

Common name: Yarrow

Family name: Compositae (Sunflower)

Botanical name: Archillea Millefolium

Other name: Gandana (Indian)

Dosha effect: P K–, V+

Taste: bitter, pungent, astringent

PD taste: pungent

Energy: cooling, drying

Actions: diaphoretic, astringent. alterative, hemostatic, vulnerary, anti-spasmodic, anti-inflammatory, tonic, antiseptic, emmenagogue, carminative

Tissues: plasma, blood, muscle

Indications: colds, fever, gastritis, enteritis, measles, menorrhagia, nosebleed, stomach ulcers, abscesses, hemoptysis, gall bladder inflammation, pelvic infection, dysmenorrhea, amenorrhea, vaginitis, wounds, varicose veins, rheumatism, headache, neuritis, hemorrhoids, gout, ambivalence, menopause, dermatitis, cellulite, acne, sunburn

Warning: sensitive skin may be irritated with exposure to sun; high Vata

YARROW (continued)

Usage: skin patches, lotion, bath, compress, massage oil

Aroma: sharp, somewhat camphoraceous odor, drying out in a sweeter, faint and pleasant note

Mixes well with: lemongrass, hyssop, clary sage, lavender, myrtle, cedarwood, angelica, St. John's wort, rosewood, citrus oils

APPENDIX A: GLOSSARY

Absolute - alcohol extracted essential oil made from concrete

Adrenals - gland producing many hormones, part of the endocrine system above each kidney

Alcohols - class of chemicals used by living organisms, which are energizing, vitalizing, anti-viral and diuretic

Aldehyde - class of chemicals used by living organisms, which have calming, sedative, anti-viral and anti-inflammatory properties

Alterative - tending to restore normal health, cleans and purifies the blood, alters existing nutritive and excretory processes, gradually restoring normal body function

Ama - Ayurvedic word for the build up of toxins

Amenorrhea - lack of menstrual period

Anthelmintic - kills intestinal worms

Antibiotic - destroys and prevents microorganisms

Antipyretic - dispels heat, fire and fever (from the Greek word pyre - fire)

Antiseptic - cleaning substance preventing development of organisms

Antispasmodic - relieves spasms of voluntary and involuntary muscles

Aphrodisiac - sexual stimulant maintains vitality, builds organs

Aromatic - plants with volatile oils

Arthritis - inflammation or swelling of the joints

Astral - "of the stars " - energy field of the body

Astringent - one of the six tastes, found in witch hazel, potatoes, beans; firms tissues and organs; reduces discharge and secretions

Aura - energy field

Auto-immune - system of body defense against foreign substances

Auto-immune disease - process where body cannot defend self, or attacks self

Ayurveda - science of life, Indian medical system

Balsamic - fragrant substance made from plant exudates that soften phlegm

Basti - medicated enema

Bile - secretion produced by the liver and stored by gall bladder, assisting digestion; emulsifies fats

Bitter - one of the six tastes found in barks, resins and tannins

Bitter tonic - bitter herbs which in small amounts stimulate digestion and otherwise help regulate lower fire in the body

Body type - blueprint, doshic predominance (Vata, Pitta, Kapha or combination)

Calming - blend of narcotic and clean-smelling essential oils (French method)

Carminative - relieves intestinal gas pain and distention; promotes peristalsis

Cellulite - inflammation of adipose (fat) tissue thought to be caused by toxin buildup

Cetones (ketones) - class of chemicals used by living organisms, having cell growth stimulation, wound healing and mucolytic (ease of flow) properties

Chakra - energy vortex on the human body connected to subtle channels and specific endocrine organs

Cholesterol - component of fat metabolic which can build up in the channels and passageways of the body; a necessary ingredient produced by the body and used in hormone production

Colic - contraction, pain in the digestive tract

Compress - cold or hot application of herbs, teas or essential oils applied to the exterior body

Concrete - sticky, waxy residue after solvent extraction of plant material

Congestion - accumulation or build up of mucous in the body

Cystitis - bladder inflammation

DNA - genetic blueprint for the entire organism, contained in every cell

Debility - lack of physical strength, weakness

Decoction - strong herbal tea concentrate

Diaphoretic - increases perspiration through the skin, releases heat from the body

Diuretic - promotes activity of kidney and bladder and increases urination

Douche - application of a mixture or solution to rinse the inside of the vagina

Dysmenorrhea - irregularity or disfunction of menstrual period

Edema - excess fluid not draining from the body

Electro-negative - physics term for substance with extra electrons

Electro-positive - physics term for substance needing electrons

Emetic - substance which induces vomiting

Emmenagogue - helps promote and regulate menstruation

Emollient - tissue-softening substance

Engorgement - congestion, blockage, enlargement

Essence - source

Esters - class of chemicals used by living organisms which are antifungal, sedative, calming, anti-spasmodic, fungicidal, balancing and anti-inflammatory

Etheric - beyond the earth - energy field of the body

Ethers - (poly-propane ethers) class of chemicals used by living organisms which are antiseptic, stimulant, expectorant, spasmolytic and diuretic

Exalting - blend of stimulating and erogenous-smelling essential oils (French method)

Expectorant - promotes discharge of phlegm and mucous from the lungs and throat

Extracted - term referring to petroleum extracted essential oils

Exudate - external plant secretion (sap, resin)

Febrifuge - substance that stops fever

Flatulence - stomach or intestinal gas

Ghee - clarified butter

Hemostatic - stops the flow of blood, a type of astringent that stops internal bleeding or hemorrhaging

Hepatic - relation to the liver

Herpes - skin eruption of viral nature

Holotropic - having to do with the whole being contained in the component parts

Hydrophilic - loves water; will combine easily with water

Hydrotherapy - water therapy

Hymoptysis - spitting or coughing blood

Hyperbaric - method of extraction using high pressure and CO_2

Hypertension - high blood pressure

Implant - holding an herb, tea, therapeutic mixture, or oil inside vagina or rectum

Infused oil - the process of steeping herbs or flowers for one or more months, then straining to obtain an oil-extracted concentrate

Inhalation - process of taking in steam and vaporized essential oils by nose or mouth

Irritant - substance aggravating body tissues

Kapha - dosha (force) composed of water and earth elements; responsible for fluids and substance in the body

Kaya Kalpa - "bodies' transformation"; process of rejuvenation which extends life for those with more work to complete on the planet

Kirlian - photos which record energy patterns or emanations from a living organism

Lactation - milk secretion

Lactones - class of chemicals used by living organisms which are an ester with a carbon ring; contain anti-inflammatory and mucolytic qualities

Laxative - promotes bowel movements

Limbic - primitive part of the brain, responsible for appetites, memories and desires

Lipophilic - loves fat or oils, will combine with them easily

Macerate - to grind

Mantle - acid covering of the skin produced by sebaceous glands; helps protect the skin

Medicated oil - produced by steeping herbs or flowers for one or more months, then straining; the same oil can be used with more plant parts to produce a 2x (double strength) oil, or 3x, etc.

Menorrhagia - excessive menstrual flow

Nervine - strengthens the functional activity of the nervous system; may be stimulants or sedatives

Neurasthenia - weakness or exhaustion of the nervous system

Nutritive - increases nutrition and tissue

Obstructed Vata - condition of excess Vata which clogs channel with toxins (ama)

PH - acid/alkaline measurement: 0-7 acid; 7 neutral; 7-14 alkaline

Pancha Karma - Ayurvedic cleansing process - seasonal body tune up

Peristalsis - rythmic, concentric, progressive, contractions of the GI tract musculature to move food mass onward

Phenols - class of chemicals used by living organisms which are strongly bactericidal, stimulant, warming, and possible skin and liver irritants

Phytoestrogen - plant estrogen

Pitta - dosha (force) in living organisms made from fire and water elements; responsible for digestion, metabolism and hormones in the body

Pituitary - master gland regulator of endocrine system

Prana - life force

Rajas (rajasic) - energy or state of working in the world; worldly, turbulent, distracting

Rasayana - Ayurvedic system of rejuvenation; herbs which slow down the aging process

Refreshing - blend of clean and stimulating-smelling essential oils (French method)

Rejuvenative - prevents decay, postpones aging, revitalizes organs

Rosin - plant sap exudate

Rubefacient - increasing circulation to the skin

Salty - one of the six tastes found in rock salt, seaweed, sea salt and vegetables

Salve - bee wax mixture with vegetable oil to preserve herbs and oils

Sattva (sattvic) - harmonious, calm, enlightened

Sedative - calms, tranquilizes, by lowering the functional activity of the organ or body part

Seer - one who sees workings of the universe through a state of connectedness

Sesquiterpenes - class of chemicals used by living organisms and having anti-inflammatory, sedative, anti-viral, anti-carcinogenic, bacteriostatic, immune stimulating, and fluid moving qualities

Shirodhara - focused stream of special oils onto the forehead, which produces calming, centering and ecstatic sensations through the nervous system

Sinusitis - irritation of sinus

Sitz bath - a therapeutic solution (tea or essential oil mix) for soaking the genitals and rectum

Sodium carbonate - salt solution used in mummification

Sour - one of the six tastes found in fats, amino acids, fermented products, vitamin C, fruits and vegetables

Stimulant - increases internal heat, dispels internal chill, strengthens metabolism and circulation

Subdosha - below, under, or a portion of the dosha (force), controlling a specific aspect of metabolism

Sultry - blend of narcotic and erogenous-smelling essential oils (French method)

Sweet - one of the six tastes found in sugar, carbohydrates, and dairy products

Tamas (tamasic) - state or mode of operation involving stagnation, stillness, darkness, dullness, resistance

Tantra - weaving of energy expansion - union, the seventh yoga

Tarpana - ancestral healing; ancient ceremony using breath and forgiveness to heal genetic tendencies

Tea - herbal beverage

Terpenes - class of chemicals used by living organisms and having stimulant, anti-viral and possible skin irritating qualities

Tincture - herbal extract using alcohol or glycerin

Tonics (nutritive) - increase weight and density and nourish the body

Vapor rub - warming mixture of herbal, vegetable and essential oils applied to the skin

Vata - dosha (force) operating in all living things, composed of the elements of ether and air, and being involved in all movements within the body

Vulnerary - assists in healing of wounds by protecting against infection and stimulating cell growth

Yang - Chinese concept of expansion, activeness, heat—positive

Yin - Chinese concept of contraction, passiveness, cool—negative

Yoni - Tantric term for vagina, meaning sacred space

APPENDIX B:
RESOURCE GUIDE

Wholesalers for Earth Essentials Oils

For information about essential oils or to send for a catalog:

For USA, except California, Oregon, Washington, Canada or Hawaii

Earth Essentials Florida, Inc.
Drs. Bryan and Light Miller
P.O. Box 35284
Sarasota, Fl. 34242
Fax (941)346-3519
Voice (941)346-3220

For California, Oregon, Washington, Canada and Hawaii

Earth Essentials California	**Lotus Light Enterprises, Inc**.
6349 Filbert Avenue	Box 1008 AA, Lotus Drive
Orangevale, CA 95662	Silver Lake, WI 53170
(916)988-4471	Fax (414)889-8951
Fax (916)988-2729	AutoFax (800) 905-6887
	Voice (800)548-3824

Wholesalers of 100% pure authentic and natural essential oils. No animals harmed or tested to produce these products.

When Purchasing Essential Oils

1. Essential oils must be protected from sunlight. Look for oils in amber or blue bottles; clear bottles could mean fragrance oils or synthetics.

2. Oils should clearly state *essential oil* on the label, and include the botanical name of the plant to avoid confusion.

3. Avoid fragrance or perfume oils (contain synthetics).

4. Oils vary in price; those which are all the same price have probably been diluted with vegetable oil (blended).

5. Follow your nose: only buy oils that smell good to you.

6. Develop your nose (discrimination) by smelling different sources of oils.

7. You get what you pay for! For instance, if rose oil is less than $75.00 for 1/4 ounce, it is blended or synthetic.

8. When possible, seek out essential oils which are organically grown, food grade, steam distilled, or cold pressed; *know your source.*

Retailers for Earth Essentials Oils

NAME	ADDRESS	CITY	STATE	ZIP
Golden Leaves Books Phone (501) 623 7007	214 Broadway	Hot Springs	AR	71901
Food for Life Herb Dept.	4747 Thomas	Phoenix	AZ	85018
Lynda Henderson (Massage)	3221 West 14th Ave.	Vancouver	BC	V6K2Y2
Healthways	4005 Manzanita Ave.	Carmichael	CA	95608
Her Place	6635 Madison Ave.	Carmichael	CA	95608
Elliotts Natural Foods	7876 Greenback Lane	Citrus Heights	CA	95610
Simply Romance	8401 Church St. Unit D	Gilroy	CA	95020
Moon Rise Herbs	981 Pine St.	Mendocino	CA	95460
Rizults	6505 Lucan Ave.	Oakland	CA	94611
Simplicity	418 Bryant Circle #G	Ojai	CA	93023

NAME	ADDRESS	CITY	STATE	ZIP
Earth Spirit	4140 Snows Road	Placerville	CA	95637
Phoenix Book Store	1120 Fulton Av. Suite H	Sacramento	CA	95825
In Harmony Herbs	4808 Santa Monica Ave.	San Diego	CA	92107
Questo Co-op	745 Francis St.	San Luis Obispo	CA	93401
Santa Barbara Nutrition Center	15 East Figuerea St.	Santa Barbara	CA	93101
Supernatural	506 State St.	Santa Barbara	CA	95101
ScentsAbilities	4397 #C Tunjunga Ave.	Studio City	CA	91604
Life Source	525 North Central Ave.	Upland	CA	91786
Stewart Mineral Springs	4617 Stewart Springs Rd.	Weed	CA	96094
TJM Sales Inc.	16251 West 74th Ave.	Arvada	CO	80007
Unitea Herbs Phone (303) 443-1248	P.O. Box 8005, #318	Boulder	CO	80306
Emerald Rose Phone (303) 938 9855	1738 Pearl St.	Boulder	CO	80302
Basic Blends Phone (303) 663 5673	428 West 1st St.	Loveland	CO	80537
D. Wilson Associates Phone (202) 526 4086	2801 Monroe St. NE	Washington	DC	20018
Teri Aldred Phone (941) 458 0337	1618 SE 2nd St.	Cape Coral	FL	33990
Therapeutic Concepts Phone (941) 337 7990	2502 2nd St. #103	Ft. Myers	FL	33901
Granary Phone (941) 366 7906	1415 Main St.	Sarasota	FL	34236
Granary Phone (941) 957 1376	1930 Stickney Point Rd.	Sarasota	FL	34231
Harmony in Mind Phone (941) 957 1376	750 South Orange	Sarasota	FL	34236
Super Value Phone (941) 366 1997	1461 Main St.	Sarasota	FL	34236
Unity Book Store Phone (941) 955 3301	800 Coconut	Sarasota	FL	34236
Mosinger Health Food Center Phone (813) 544 5060	6531 54th Av. North	St. Petersburg	FL	33709
Gecko Trading Co.	3621 Baldwin Ave.	Makawao	HI	96768
North Shore Silks	P.O. Box 1416	Paia, Maui	HI	96779
Life Spring	3178 North Clark St.	Chicago	IL	60657

Essentials Oils Retailers (continued)

NAME	ADDRESS	CITY	STATE	ZIP
Alternative Health Services Phone (410) 257 3735	4521 Chavez Court	Chesapeake Beach	MD	20732
Health Concern Phone (410) 828 4015	28 W. Susquehana Ave.	Towson	MD	21204
Apple Valley Phone (616) 394 1445	12360 Felch St.	Holland	MI	49424
Uncommon Scents & Gifts Phone (517) 839 6600	150 East Main St.	Midland	MI	48640
Say Yes to Life Phone (417) 679 4145	305 North Main St.	Gainesville	MO	65655
Celestial Horizons, Inc. Phone (417) 889 9940	5337 F So. Campbell St.	Springfield	MO	65810
Renaissance Book & Gift Phone (417) 883 5167	1337 East Montclair	Springfield	MO	65804
Moonrise Herbs Phone (707) 937 1146	18th and Bay View	Barnegat	NJ	08006
Cid's Natural Foods Phone (505) 758 1148	822 Paseo Del Pueblo Norte	El Prado	NM	87529
Iris Herbal Products Phone (505) 988 8961	3204 HWY 522	San Cristobal	NM	87564
Body Therapy Phone (505) 984 1879	1004 Don Albero Ave.	Santa Fe	NM	87501
Herbs, Etc. Phone (505) 984 3208	323 Aztec	Santa Fe	NM	87501
Vitality Unlimited Phone (505) 983 5557	513 Camino de los Marquez	Santa Fe	NM	87501
Wild Oats Market Phone (505) 983 5333	1090 St. Francis Dr.	Santa Fe	NM	87501
Crystal Center Phone (505) 751 0959	114 La Dona Luz	Taos	NM	87571
Merlin's Garden Phone (505) 758 0985	127 A Bent St.	Taos	NM	87571
Silver Sage	157 South Virginia St.	Reno	NV	89503
Contours Beauty Spa Phone (716) 225-2130	2300 Ridge Road West	Rochester	NY	14626
Antrican	304 East 13th Ave.	Eugene	OR	97401
Virginia's Gifts & Herbs	236 Garibaldi Ave.	Garibaldi	OR	97178
Lawson's Aromatics Phone (717) 252 3990	409 Cherry St.	Wrightsville	PA	17868

NAME	ADDRESS	CITY	STATE	ZIP
Kathy's Ranch	4695 So. Holliday Blvd.	Salt Lake City	UT	84117
Vincent Munden Phone(703) 715 0256	13100 Thompson Rd.	Fairfax	VA	22033
Grace Place Store Phone (804) 359 1183	826 West Grace St.	Richmond	VA	23220
Heritage Store, Inc. Phone (804) 428 0500	314 Laskin Rd.	Virginia Beach	VA	23451
All About Beauty Phone (304) 442-0082	201 W Washington St.	Lewisburg	WV	24901

Ayurvedic Studies

American Institute of Vedic Studies
P.O. Box 8357
Santa Fe, NM 87501
(505) 983-9385
Correspondence Course in
Ayurveda by Dr. David Frawley

Ayurvedic Healing Arts Center
16508 Pine Knoll Rd.
Grass Valley, CA 95945
(916) 274-9000

Ayurvedic Institute
& Wellness Center
P.O. Box 23445
Albuquerque, NM 87192-1445
(505) 291-9698
Correspondence Course "Lessons
and Lectures in Ayurveda" by Dr.
Robert E. Svoboda

Himalayan Institute
RR1, Box 400
Honesdale, PA 18431
(800) 822-4547

Earth Essentials Florida
5415 Cape Layte Dr.
Sarasota, FL 34242
(941) 346-3220

Institute for Wholistic Education
33719 116th St., Box AA
Twin Lakes, WI 53181
(414) 889-8501
Correspondence Course in
Ayurveda

Lotus Ayurvedic Center
4145 Clares Street, Suite D
Capitola, CA 95010

Aromatherapy Studies

Canadian Federation of Aromatherapy
P.O. Box 68571-1235
Williams Parkway East
Bramalea, Ontario L6S6A1
(905) 457-6711

Jeanne Rose
219 Carl Street
San Francisco, CA 94117
(415) 564-6799
Aromatherapy and herbal home study course, essential oils, hydrolates

Kurt Schnaubelt
P.O. Box 606
San Rafael, CA 94915

The National Association
for Holistic Aromatherapy
P.O. Box 17622
Boulder, CO 80308

Ayurvedic Treatment Centers

Ayurveda at Spirit Rest
P.O. Box 3537
Pagosa Springs, CO 81147-3537
(970) 264-2573

Ayurvedic Institute
& Wellness Center
P.O. Box 23445
Albuquerque, NM 87192-1445
(505) 291-9698

Center for Mind, Body Medicine
P.O. Box 1048
La Jolla, CA 92038
(619) 794-2425

Diamond Way Health Associates
214 Girard Boulevard, N.E.
Albuquerque, NM 87106
(505) 265-4826

Earth Essentials Florida
5415 Cape Layte Dr.
Sarasota, FL 34242
(941) 346-3220

Integrated Health Systems
3855 Via Nova Marie, #302D
Carmel, CA 93923
(408) 476-5130

Kaya Kalpa International
Dr. Raam Panday
111 Woodster Road
Satto, NY 10012
(212) 925-8272

Dr. Lobsang Rapgay
2206 Benecia Avenue
West Los Angeles, CA 90064)
(310) 282-9918

Ayurvedic Treatment Centers (continued)

Lotus Ayurvedic Center
4145 Clares Street, Suite D
Capitola, CA 95010
(408) 479-1667

Wise Earth Foundation
Bri. Maya Tiwari
25 Howland Road, #R8
Asheville, North Carolina 28804
(704) 258-9999
(Re-opens Spring 1996, for Teachers and
Practitioners Training Programs only.)

Ayurvedic Herbal Suppliers

Auroma International
P.O. Box 1008-AA
Silver Lake, WI 53170
(414) 889-8569

Ayur Herbal Corporation
P.O. Box 6390-AA
Santa Fe, NM 87502
(414) 889-8569

Ayurveda Center of Santa Fe
1807 Second St., Suite 20
Santa Fe, NM 87505
(505) 983-8898

Ayurvedic Institute
& Wellness Center
11311 Menaul N.E., Suite A
Albuquerque, NM 87112
(505) 291-9698

Ayush Herbs Inc.
10025 N.E. 4th Street
Bellevue, WA 98004
(800) 925-1371

Bazaar of India Imports, Inc.
1810 University Avenue
Berkley, CA 94703
(800) 261-7662

Earth Essentials Florida
5415 Cape Layte Dr.
Sarasota, FL 34242
(941) 346-3220

Frontier Herbs
P.O. Box 229
Norway, Iowa 52318
(800) 669-3275

Kanak
P.O. Box 13653
Albuquerque, NM 87192-3653
(505) 275-2469

Khenpa Co.
Ayurvedic Beauty Products
17595 Harvard, Suite C-531
Irvine, CA 92714
(714) 778-0222

Ayurvedic Herbal Suppliers (continued)

Lotus Brands, Inc.
P.O. Box 325-AA
Twin Lakes, WI 53181
(262) 889-8561

Lotus Light
P.O. Box 1008-AA
Silver Lake, WI 53170
(262) 889-8501

Lotus Ayurvedic Center
4145 Clares Street, Suite D
Capitola, CA 95010
(408) 479-1667

Tej Beauty Enterprises, Inc.
162 West 56th Street, Room 201
New York, NY 10019
(212) 581-8136

Internatural
33719 116th St.
Twin Lakes, WI 53181
(262) 889-8581 or 800-643-4221
www.internatural.com
Retail Mail Order Supplier of
Ayurvedic Books, Herbal Products,
Essential Oils & Personal Care Items

**The resources and suppliers listed in this guide
are not necessarily endorsed by the authors.**

BIBLIOGRAPHY

AROMATHERAPY

Arctander, Steffen. *Perfume and Flavor Materials of Natural Origin.* Det Hoffensbergske Ettablissement: Denmark, 1960.

Berwick, Ann. *Holistic Aromatherapy: Balance the Mind and the Soul With Essential Oils.* Llewellyn Publications: St. Paul, Minnesota, 1994.

England, Allison. *Aromatherapy for Mother and Baby.* Healing Arts Press: Rochester, Vermont, 1994.

Fischer-Rizzi, Susanne. *Complete Aromatherapy Handbook: Essential Oils for Radiant Health.* Sterling Publishing Co.: New York, 1990.

Lavabre, Marcel. *Aromatherapy Workbook.* Healing Arts Press: Rochester, Vermont, 1990.

Miller, Richard Allen and Iona. *The Magical and Ritual Use of Perfumes.* Destiny Books: Rochester, Vermont, 1990.

Price, Shirley. *Aromatherapy for Common Ailments.* Simon and Schuster, Inc.: New York, 1991.

Price, Shirley. *Practical Aromatherapy: How to Use Essential Oils to Restore Vitality.* Thorsons Publishing Group: England, 1987.

Rose, Jeanne. *The Aromatherapy Book.* North Atlantic Books: Berkeley, CA, 1992.

Ryman, Daniéle. *The Aromatherapy Handbook: The Secret Healing Powers of Essential Oils.* The C.W. Daniel Company Limited: London, 1984.

Schnaubelt, Dr. Kurt. *Aromatherapy Correspondence Course.* San Rafael, CA, 1985.

Tisserand, Maggie. *Aromatherapy for Women.* Thorsons Publishers, Inc.: New York, 1985.

Tisserand, Robert. *Aromatherapy: To Heal and Tend the Body.* Lotus Press: Twin Lakes, Wisconsin, 1988.

Tisserand, Robert B. *The Art of Aromatherapy.* Destiny Books, Rochester, Vermont, 1977.

Tisserand, Robert. *The Essential Oil Safety Data Manual..* The Tisserand Aromatherapy Institute: England, 1990.

Valnet, Jean, M.D. *The Practice of Aromatherapy.* Healing Arts Press: Rochester, Vermont, 1990.

Worwood, Valerie Ann. *The Complete Book of Essential Oils and Aromatherapy.* New World Library: San Rafael, CA, 1991.

HERBOLOGY AND OTHERS

Anand, Margo. *The Art of Sexual Ecstasy.* Jeremy P. Tarcher, Inc.: Los Angeles, CA, 1989.

Chopra, Dr. Deepak. *Quantum Healing: Exploring the Frontiers of Mind/Body Medicine.* Bantam Books: New York, NY, 1989.

Green, James. *The Male Herbal: Health Care for Men and Boys.* The Crossing Press: Freedom, CA, 1991.

Johari, Harish. *Ancient Indian Massage.* Munshiram Manoharlal Publishers: New Delhi, 1984.

Leadbeater, C.W. *The Chakras.* The Theosophical Publishing House: Wheaton, IL, 1990.

Tierra, Michael, C.A, N.D. *The Way of Herbs.* Unity Press: Santa Cruz, CA, 1980.

Weed, Susan S. *Menopausal Years: The Wise Woman Way.* Ash Tree Publishing: Woodstock, NY, 1992.

AYURVEDA

American Institute of Vedic Studies. *Ayurvedic Study Course.* Santa Fe, NM.

Chopra, Dr. Deepak. *Perfect Health.* Harmony Books: New York, 1991.

Dash, Vaidya Bhagwan and Junius, Acarya, Manfred M. *A Hand Book of Ayurveda.* Concept Publishing Company: New Delhi, 1983.

Frawley, Dr. David. *Ayurvedic Healing, a Comprehensive Guide.* Passage Press: Salt Lake City, Utah, 1989.

Frawley, Dr. David and Lad, Dr. Vasant. *The Yoga of Herbs, An Ayurvedic Guide to Herbal Medicine.* Lotus Press: Twin Lakes, WI, 1986.

Garde, Dr. R. K. *Ayurveda for Health and Long Life.* D. B. Taraporevala Sons and Co. Private Ltd.: Bombay, India, 1975.

Heyn, Birgit. *Ayurvedic Medicine.* Thorsons Publishing Group: Wellingborough, Northamptonshire, England, 1987.

Lad, Dr. Vasant. *Ayurveda, The Science of Self-Healing, A Practical Guide.* Lotus Press: Twin Lakes, WI, 1984.

Maharishi Ayur-Ved Medical Association. *Maharishi Ayur-Veda Physician Training Course I: Phase I and Phase II.* Maharishi Ayur Veda Foundation, 1993.

Ojha, Divalar and Kumar, Ashok. *Panchakarma-Therapy in Ayurveda, Chaukhamba Amarabharati Studies Vol. VI.* Chaukhamba Amarabharati Prakashan Publishers: Varanasi, India, 1978.

Sachs, Melanie. *Ayurvedic Beauty Care, Ageless Techniques to Invoke Natural Beauty.* Lotus Press: Twin Lakes, WI, 1994.

Sharma, P.V. *Caraka Samhita, Volumes I, II, and III.* Chaukhambha Orientalia: Varanasi, Delhi, India, 1992.

Svoboda, Dr. Robert E. *Ayurveda: Life, Health and Longevity.* Penguin Books: London, England, 1992.

Svoboda, Dr. Robert E. *Prakruti, Your Ayurvedic Constitution.* Geocom Limited, Albuquerque, NM, 1988.

INDEX

elements
  five element theory, 11
  and taste, 35-38
elemi, 250
emesis, 205
emetic, 84
emmenagogue, 84, 96
  cooling, for Kapha, 107
  cooling, for Pitta, 101
  heating, for Kapha, 107
  for Vata, 96
emollient, 84
emotions, 29, 165-169
  essential oils to use when feeling:
    absentminded, 168; angry, 168;
    attached, 169; depressed, 169;
    disinterested, 169; domineering,
    168; fearful, 167; frustrated, 168;
    greedy, 169; hurtful, 168;
    irritable, 169; moody, 168;
    opinionated, 168; ; resistant,
    169; sad, 169; scattered, un-
    grounded, 167; sleepless, 168;
    stubborn, 168;
    uncertain, 169; unfocused, 168;
    weak, 168
  patterns of, 167
  See also body type questionnaire
endocrine organs, 162-163
enema (basti), 202
environmental fragrancing, 131
essential oils, 75
  absolute, 78
  affects on the body, 79-81
  care and selection of, 78
  cold pressing, 77
  concrete, 78
  for Kapha imbalance, 103
  for Pitta imbalance, 99

  for Vata imbalance, 94
  production of, 76
    CO_2 hyperbaric method, 77
    solvent extraction method, 77
    steam distillation, 70, 76
  See also oil families
esters, 90
ether, 12
ethers, 91
eucalyptus, 251
exercise, 149
expectorant, 84
  for Kapha, 107

F

fennel, 253
  cooking with, 136
fever
  inhalation for, 123
fir, 254
fire, 12
flax oil, 118
flu
  inhalation for, 123
frankinsence, 255
Frawley, David, 84, 93, 155, 220

G

galbanum, 310
gall bladder, 158
garlic, 256
Gattefosse, Dr. Rene-Maurice, 72
gemstones, 195-199
  agate, 195
  amber, 195

Pitta, 142
Vata, 142
nosebleed during, 143
poor circulation during, 144
stretch marks, 142
toothache during, 143
varicose veins during, 144
primrose oil, 120
pulse, 30-33
pungent, 37
purgation (virechana), 201

R

rajas, 166
See also mind
rasayana, 210
rejuvenative, 85
for Kapha, 107
for Pitta, 101
Rishis, 8
rose, 285
rosemary, 287
cooking with, 137
rosewood, 288

S

safflower oil, 119
saffron, 325
sage, 289
cooking with, 137
St. Johns wort, 326
salty, 36
salves, 129
sandalwood, 290

sattva, 167
See also mind
savory, 327
seaweed, 328
sedative, 85
sesame oil, 118
sesquiterpenes, 90
shamama, 329
shirodhara, 206
sinusitis
inhalation for, 123
skin care, 125
for Kapha, 128
for Pitta, 127
for Vata, 127
smell, 67
See also olfactory nerve
snehana
See oelation
sour, 36
soy oil, 119
spirit, 161-165
stimulant, 85
for Kapha, 105
for Vata, 98
stomach
complaints, 156
styrax, 329
subdoshas, 39-52
Alochaka Pitta, 46
Apana Vata, 42
Avalambaka Kapha, 48
Bhrajaka Pitta, 46
Bodhaka Kapha, 47
Kledaka Kapha, 48
Pachaka Pitta, 44
Prana Vata, 40

ABOUT THE AUTHORS

As a child, Dr. Light Miller, or Jyoti (her Indian name), traveled all over the world learning and assimilating the natural ways of living in many cultures. Her East Indian background gives her a strong connection to her roots in Ayurveda, which she learned from her Grandmother, who practiced with Ayurvedic herbs. Her mother introduced her to the uses of essential oils and herbal products for skin care. Her familiarity with tropical flowers and herbs comes from time spent in the Caribbean.

In 1968, Light graduated from the University of California, Berkeley, and shortly thereafter graduated from the Los Angeles School of Massage, where she felt her calling as a healer. This experience awakened her natural interest in meditation, yoga and Eastern philosophy. She has 25 years' experience as a health practitioner, and has trained over 700 people in the field of massage.

Currently, Light provides individual Ayurvedic counseling, and is the first woman in the world to practice Kaya Kalpa. She received training from Dr. Raam Panday of New York, and a 110-year-young master, Dr. Chotay, in India.

Light is working on her next book, about women's awakening power through the goddesses of Indian mythology.

Dr. Bryan Miller, D.C., received his Chiropractic Degree from Western States Chiropractic College in 1979. He practiced holistic medicine in California and Hawaii, integrating bodywork, herbology, diet and emotional release work. Dr. Miller travels around the world teaching Cross Fiber Massage, Tantra, Aromatherapy, and Ayurveda, and providing specialized treatments. An avid outdoor enthusiast, he enjoys hiking, surfing, diving, and sport fishing. He is one of 18 Kaya Kalpa practitioners in the world.

During the summer, Bryan and Light enjoy international travel, teaching courses in Aromatherapy, Ayurveda, Natural Menopause, Herbology, and Tantra. In the fall and winter, Light and Bryan live in Florida where they conduct Pancha Karma programs and Kaya Kalpa treatments. They also teach a Rasayana (rejuvenation) program: an eight-week residential intensive that covers advanced techniques in Ayurveda and holistic healing. Their company, Earth Essentials, distributes high-quality essential oils and other related products.

For information regarding treatment programs, seminars or lectures, you may write or call:

EARTH ESSENTIALS

P.O. BOX 35284
Sarasota, FL 34242
Voice: (941) 346-3220
Fax: (941) 346-3519

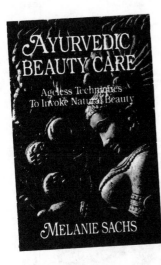

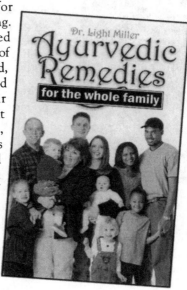